Sustainable Food:

How to Buy Right and Spend Less

ELISE McDONOUGH

Chelsea Green Publishing
White River Junction, Vermont

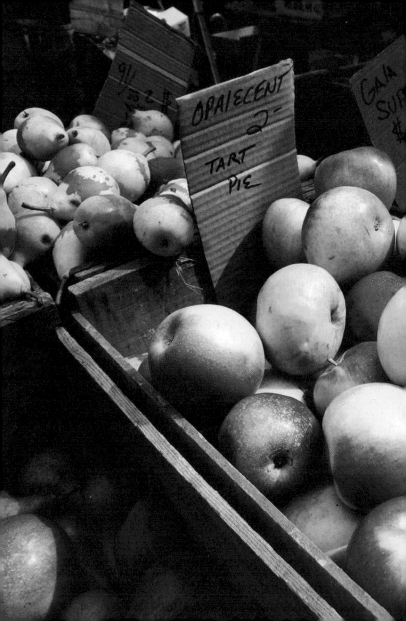

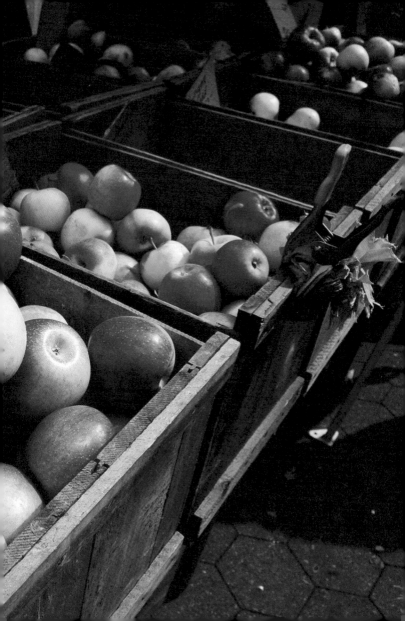

Project Manager: Patricia Stone
Developmental Editor: Ben Watson
Copy Editor: Cannon Labrie
Proofreader: Helen Walden

Printed in Canada
First printing August, 2009
10 9 8 7 6 5 4 3 2 1   09 10 11 12 13

Our Commitment to Green Publishing
Chelsea Green sees publishing as a tool for cultural change and ecological stewardship. We strive to
align our book manufacturing practices with our editorial mission and to reduce the impact of our
business enterprise in the environment. We print our books and catalogs on chlorine-free recycled
paper, using vegetable-based inks whenever possible. This book may cost slightly more because we
use recycled paper, and we hope you'll agree that it's worth it. Chelsea Green is a member of the
Green Press Initiative (www.greenpressinitiative.org), a nonprofit coalition of publishers, manufactur-
ers, and authors working to protect the world's endangered forests and conserve natural resources.
Sustainable Food was printed on Silva Enviro, a 100-percent postconsumer recycled paper supplied
by Marquis.

Library of Congress Cataloging-in-Publication Data
McDonough, Elise, 1980-
  Sustainable food : how to buy right and spend less / Elise McDonough.
      p. cm.
  Includes bibliographical references.
  ISBN 978-1-60358-141-7
  1. Natural foods. 2. Grocery shopping. 3. Sustainable living. I. Title.

  TX369.M42 2009
  641.3'02--dc22

                              2009019576

Chelsea Green Publishing Company
Post Office Box 428
White River Junction, VT 05001
(802) 295-6300
www.chelseagreen.com

CONTENTS

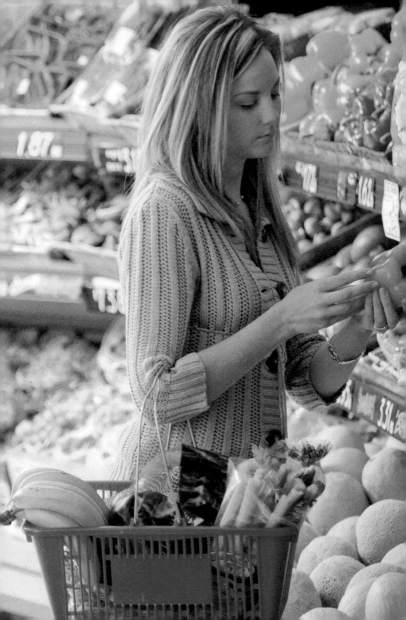

AN INTRODUCTION TO ETHICAL EATING

Food embodies the most basic connection human beings share with each other and the earth. Choosing sustainable ways of feeding ourselves, by changing how we shop, cook, eat, and drink, means helping to save the planet, three times a day or more. And remember, eating "green" is healthier, fresher, and tastier than the fast-food alternative, so your taste buds will definitely benefit along with the environment.

In terms of fighting global climate change, simply eating less meat and buying local produce makes more of a positive contribution than ditching your gas-guzzling SUV for a hybrid electric car. If everyone in the United States adopted a wholly vegetarian diet (or limited meat consumption to just three or four days a week), we would greatly reduce our consumption of fossil fuels, not to mention eliminate much of the need for pollution and energy-intensive "factory farming."

Prior to the Industrial Revolution, most people either produced their own food or knew the person who did. No one had to question where dinner came from, whether or not it was safe to eat, or if one were unwittingly harming the environment in producing it. Ever since the rapid changes in the world's agricultural-production methods that followed World War II, however—when we moved from a largely local, organic, sustainable system to a globalized, chemically based, unsustainable one—a dedicated ethical eating movement has been trying to warn us about the dangers of industrial food production.

Yet only now have mainstream food consumers begun to understand that fulfilling our most basic human need often links us to the fuel-guzzling distribution methods of the nationwide grocery chains, the cruel factory-farming practices of corporate meat production, and the pesticide pollution inherent in modern agribusiness techniques. Also, many people have come to recognize that the relatively cheap products in the grocery store actually have hidden costs, such as the degradation of the environment and the epidemic of diabetes and obesity in our children.

When confronted by the dizzying array of up to 40,000 products in the average U.S. supermarket, it can be difficult and time-consuming to consider how any one item either supports or clashes with your ideals. But after educating yourself on the issues, you can create your own hierarchy of food choices to serve as a guide, one that reflects the issues you feel most passionate about. For instance, if you care deeply about shielding your family from the ill effects of pesticide residues, then organic products will rise to the top of your shopping list. If you want to protect local farmers from the encroachment of corporate competitors and housing developments, then "vote with your fork" and select local, seasonal produce: You'll not only experience the variety of sensory delights found in each season; you'll also save money by avoiding expensive, exotic food flown in from distant lands.

Seven Simple Considerations

The basic hierarchy followed in this book, inspired by the Natural Gourmet Institute's founder, Annemarie Colbin, is *whole*, *seasonal*, *organic*, *local*, *fresh*, *real*, and *delicious*. Let's start our edible adventure by defining each of these terms.

Whole
Whole foods exist as close to their natural state as possible, and rep-

resent the simplest and most nutritious form of human sustenance. Increasing the amount of whole foods in your diet will instantly cut down on the amount of unhealthy additives you consume, while simultaneously reducing your carbon footprint.

Whole foods arrive in their natural packaging, such as a peel or skin, which can easily be composted, along with inedible cores, seeds, or stems, thus reducing the amount of household garbage that ends up in a landfill. More importantly, by avoiding processed foods, you opt out of an industrial food-production system that converts *whole*some ears of corn into industrial products like high-fructose corn syrup, and that considers synthetic food additives like aspartame, monosodium glutamate, and trans fats to be part of a balanced diet.

Grains are whole foods when they are minimally processed (brown rice, oat groats, wheat berries, etc). Fruit must have no edible pieces removed. For instance, apples are whole foods, but apple juice is not. In the kitchen, meals that are created from whole ingredients are considered "wholesome." For example, a smoothie blended together from berries, bananas, cashews, and whole milk can be considered a whole food, since all of the ingredients qualify.

It's easy to find whole foods in the produce section, bakery, deli, or dairy case on the periphery of your grocery store, whereas heavily processed, "packaged goods" typically rule the center aisles. When you must venture into the center of the labyrinth, consider leaving your cart behind, to discourage impulse buys.

Seasonal
Seasonal foods arrive in abundance at a particular time of year, such as pumpkins in the autumn, parsnips in the winter, asparagus in the spring, and strawberries in the summer. Adding seasonal foods to your own diet means challenging your palate with new dishes and connecting your kitchen to the larger rhythms of the planet.

Before our modern system of shipping and refrigeration, almost all food was seasonal, and you'll definitely find this reflected in traditional recipes. For instance, *pasta primavera* translates as "springtime pasta," and includes vegetables like fresh peas that ripen at that time of year. And while making roasted asparagus in the winter sounds like a delicious idea too, it's less so when you consider all the extra fuel required to airfreight those tender spears from South America. Better to wait till spring and buy local.

Seasonal eaters also save money and get fresher food, since they buy perishable items when they are most abundant. To extend the season, you can preserve some of this bounty through methods of food storage like canning, pickling, drying, and freezing. Small-scale home canning and freezing efforts are much more energy efficient than industrial processing, once you take into account the energy required to transport these foods to your local supermarket, and from there to your pantry or home freezer.

Organic

Organic foods, including fruits, vegetables, grains, meat, milk, and cheeses, have been produced without the use of chemical pesticides or synthetic fertilizers. Removing these largely petroleum-based inputs from the food chain fights global warming, reverses soil degradation, and produces healthier, more sustainable foods. The USDA also rejects genetically modified organisms (GMOs) when awarding organic certification.

Originally, the organic farming movement sought not only to avoid synthetic fertilizers and pesticides, but also to address the myriad other drawbacks of industrialized agriculture by supporting small, diverse, local, and eco-friendly food producers. However, the success of organic products in the marketplace has attracted large corporate investment and government interference, both of which continue to transform the movement. It's important to remember that, while the

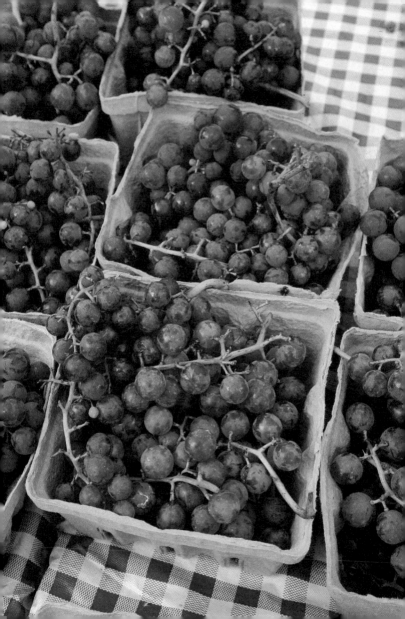

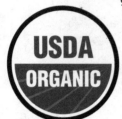

greater availability of certified organic products represents a victory for consumers, the struggle to secure safe, sustainable food for everyone remains far from over. One way you can help is to join the Organic Consumers Association, and help fight the agrochemical companies and corporate agribusinesses that constantly lobby the USDA to weaken existing organic standards.

Meanwhile, despite their recent, rapid growth, organics still constitute a very small sector of the overall food economy. Also, as just mentioned, large corporations have muscled in on this increasingly profitable market. On the plus side this means less pesticide pollution, and more accessibility and affordability for consumers; on the minus side it usually means a continuation of agribusiness as usual, such as factory-style, monocrop farming, and the long-distance transportation of organic produce from remote locales to markets.

According to the USDA, anything labeled "100% Organic" must contain less than 5 percent nonorganic material, while the "organic" label mandates at least 90 percent organic ingredients, and "Made with Organic Ingredients" requires 70 percent organic ingredients. Organic produce can have some pesticide residue on it, according to a 2002 Consumers Union report. While detectable residues were much lower compared to conventional items, some organic items can be tainted by pesticide drift from neighboring nonorganic farms. And organic meat or poultry may, in some circumstances, have been fed a certain amount of nonorganic grain or hay, or the animals treated, if sick, with antibiotics. When antibiotics are used on an animal it is removed from the herd and not reunited until all drugs are out of its system. In the case of organic dairy cows on antibiotics, their milk is not added to the food supply until they are healthy again.

Local

The commonly accepted standard for local food means it was grown, gathered, hunted, or raised within a 100-mile radius of where you live. Self-described "locavores" refer to this area as their "foodshed." A consumer's dietary impact on the ecosystem is referred to as the "foodprint," a riff on the popular "footprint" metaphor that measures an individual's overall carbon impact based on their lifestyle. Purchasing local foods directly supports small-scale farms, giving the farmer more of your grocery dollar and keeping money circulating within the local economy.

Throwing a 100-mile dinner party offers a fun way to learn about the bounty of your own foodshed, while simultaneously spreading the word about the benefits of local eating, including freshness, value, reduction of energy consumption, and support for nearby farmers.

Fresh

For optimal taste and nutrition, fresh food should be eaten as soon as possible after it has been picked, harvested, caught, or slaughtered. Avoid using frozen and canned foods whenever possible. Frozen foods consume tons of energy in order to stay below freezing until you're ready to cook them. Canned foods are convenient and have a long shelf life, but they also rely on an energy-intensive production process.

Instead, when fresh food is not available or preferable, investigate traditional methods of food preservation—like drying, pickling, and fermenting—that can actually make food healthier! While canning and freezing foods requires energy, it's still more efficient to preserve food at home with these methods if driving to the store to buy prepackaged frozen food is the alternative. "Putting food by" is a traditional and valuable skill for thrifty and eco-conscious families.

Real

A Twinkie is a tangible item. It can be seen, touched, and tasted. So is it *real*? For the purposes of this discussion, it is not. "Real" food, in our definition of the term, will exclude any product of industrial refining processes, excluding not just junk food and fast food, but many of the packaged goods found in the modern supermarket—everything from what Gorton's calls "fish sticks" to what Kraft calls "macaroni and cheese." Those fake foods aren't grown or even cooked like "real" foods: they're imagined into being by a corporate marketing team, created in a lab by a food scientist, constructed out of refined ingredients, artificial flavors, and preservatives, and then heavily promoted and advertised.

The famous question organic farmers posed to the USDA certification program is "Can a Twinkie be organic?" Well yes, technically, because Hostess could start with organic ingredients and then highly refine or process them. But in many ways the concept of organic "convenience" foods is antithetical to the true spirit of the original organic-foods movement. So look beyond the label and don't assume that highly processed "organic foods" (of which there are many) are good for us or for the planet.

Delicious

Eating right for the planet isn't about deprivation: it's about gaining a new perspective on food and a better understanding of the role humanity plays in the greater ecosystem. The experience of cooking and eating should be one of life's great joys, not a chore to dread or a routine to take for granted. Be mindful of tastes, and know that real, whole, fresh, local, seasonal organic food should be delicious food too!

Savor your food, chew thoroughly, and make time to eat without distractions. Appreciate the colors, textures, and beautiful forms of fruits and vegetables. Eating slowly brings increased satisfaction, and dining purposefully with good intentions makes food that much more pleasurable.

What's That Mean?

A few other terms you may hear while navigating the marketplace.

Biodynamic

Fruit, veggies, herbs, honey, wine . . . just about anything can be produced biodynamically, with stellar results. Biodynamics grew from a series of lectures that Austrian philosopher Rudolf Steiner gave to an audience of farmers in 1924. Not only does the method prohibit the use of synthetic fertilizers, pesticides, and herbicides, but the recipes for Steiner's alternative preparations sometimes read like a witch's spell, in one case instructing that manure be stuffed into a cow's horn and buried for up to a year, then unearthed and used to create a composted manure tea.

Extensive use of lunar and astrological planting calendars encourages further cosmic vitality to be imparted to the food. Practitioners report outstanding results in quality as well as soil health.

Conventional Foods

Instead of calling the current system "industrial, chemical, polluting, unsustainable agriculture," the word "conventional" is most often applied to the huge, corporate-run agribusiness model of food production. Conventional farms use synthetic fertilizers and toxic pesticides, herbicides, and fungicides. They're dependent on heavy machinery, petroleum, monocropping, and government subsidies.

By the way, the first definition of "conventional" in the dictionary reads, "conforming to socially accepted customs of behavior or style, especially in a way that lacks imagination," and this indeed is true of conventional farming. What needs changing is our tacit social acceptance of a system of feeding ourselves that destroys the very earth we depend on.

Genetically modified organisms

Genetically modified organisms (GMOs) have caused controversy since their introduction. Advocates for GMOs argue that by altering one gene in a food crop, it's possible to greatly reduce or completely eliminate use of harmful pesticides, herbicides, or fungicides, as well as increasing productivity and saving lives in Third World countries. Mainly, however, crop plants are modified for practical but lackluster reasons, such as to make them tougher in order to withstand long-distance shipping. Modification has never been about increasing flavor—in fact, it usually does the opposite. GMO tomatoes might be able to weather a trip from San Diego to Boston, but they arrive tasting as bland as wet paper.

Mainstream environmentalists are generally anti-GMO, arguing that lack of research on these crops has potentially introduced dangerous new organisms into our world. Outrage over the patenting of GMO crops, the introduction of a "Terminator" gene that destroys the fertility of seeds from one year's crop to the next, and the drifting of GMO pollen onto non-GMO crops have turned people against genetic modification and the corporations that promote it. Public opposition has thus far led the USDA to prohibit any GMO crops or livestock from being certified under the Organic Foods Production Act.

Local versus Organic

When confronted with the dilemma of choosing between a local, conventional food and an imported, organic one, you'll have to follow your gut (not to mention your stomach), because it's impossible to give one definitive answer to a question with so many potential variables. You may feel best about choosing whatever costs less,

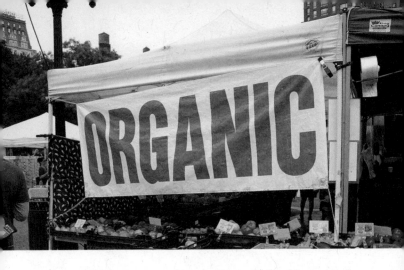

whatever's healthiest for you, whatever's best for local farmers, whatever helps reduce global warming, whatever tastes best, or finding some middle ground among all of these worthy (and sometimes competing) goals.

In many ways, organic versus local represents a false choice. Pesticide-free food shouldn't be a luxury or a privilege reserved for the well-to-do, and we should all live in communities that support and value local farming. Unfortunately, under our current system, taxpayers subsidize industrial mega-farms that produce conventional crops to the tune of tens of billions of dollars per year, creating a surplus of artificially cheap, toxic food that pollutes the soil, air, and water. Meanwhile, almost no government money goes to help small farmers transition to organic production, and these local, diversified food producers constantly face the danger of going out of business.

Conscientious consumers and other concerned citizens need to act decisively to ensure that in the future our tax dollars benefit organic, local, environmentally benign farming. Subsidizing sustainable farms would immediately bring the price of locally grown organic meats, dairy, and produce down tremendously, making them more afford-able for everyone. Changing these policies is the key to reversing the destructive agricultural trends of the past sixty years.

Shopping

A few tips to help you save money and make shopping for food easier, greener, and more efficient.

Getting to and fro

Organize your food shopping carefully, and you'll save time and money and conserve fossil fuels. Keep an updated shopping list on the refrig-

ALTERNATIVE DIETS DEFINED

Vegetarian. *Generally, vegetarians do not eat meat of any type, including fish. Some vegetarians eat eggs, some use dairy products, while still others eat neither.*

Pescetarian. *Pescetarians eat fish, but not any other animal flesh.*

Vegan. *Vegans do not consume, use, or wear any type of animal product, including meat, eggs, dairy, honey, gelatin, and leather.*

Flexitarian. *Flexitarians eat meat rarely, reserving it for special occasions or cultural exceptions.*

Raw foodist. *Raw foodists focus on eating raw fruits, veggies, and nuts, based on a belief that heating foods above 118°F (48°C) destroys much of their nutritional value.*

Freegan. *Freegans eat discarded foodstuffs from dumpsters or otherwise locate free sources of safe, edible, unwanted food that would otherwise go to waste.*

erator, and consider planning a week's worth of meals in advance to avoid driving to the market for just a few items. Not only will you make fewer, more efficient shopping trips, you'll also avoid costly impulse buys that eat away at your budget. Carpooling to the market with a friend saves even more fuel, and makes shopping a lot more fun!

B.Y.O.B. (Bring your own bags and bottles)

Plastic shows up everywhere in our daily lives, from individually wrapped slices of cheese to shopping bags and water bottles that are typically discarded after only one use. The waste and pollution associated with plastic items threatens all forms of life, in many different ways, so reduce, reuse, and recycle plastic aggressively—in that order of importance.

Locavore. These are adventurous souls who emphasize eating locally grown foods, often defining "local" as coming from within a 100-mile range. This varies in difficulty based on where you reside. A locavore in California's San Joaquin Valley might have almonds, avocados, and citrus virtually within arm's reach, year-round, while one in Portland, Maine, might enjoy fiddle-head ferns in spring and wild blueberries during summer, but would be largely restricted to storage crops like potatoes, dried beans, and squash in the winter. Omnivores may be able to eat locally with more ease than vegetarians, but a full knowledge of food preservation can ensure any local eater a reasonably diverse diet throughout the winter.

Macrobiotic. Developed by a Japanese doctor and called the "long life" diet, macrobiotic eating is low in fat and high in fiber. It is a favored approach among many people who have serious health problems, but can be too restrictive for most others. The diet consists of whole grains, lots of miso soup, plenty of raw veggies, beans, seaweed, and local fruit, as well as small amounts of seafood and nuts.

The plastic menace begins during manufacturing, a petroleum-fueled operation that releases toxic chemicals into the air, land, and water. Plastic also does not biodegrade, so your bags and bottles will be in existence for hundreds, if not thousands, of years.

Americans discard about 100 billion plastic bags each year. Those that don't make it to landfills float along on gusts of wind instead, until they get caught in a tree or end up in a lake or river. Once these bags reach the ocean, they can be mistaken for food by marine critters, poisoning them or blocking their digestive tracts. Ocean currents also collect plastics in vast floating wastelands, like the so-called garbage patch, larger than the state of Texas, that's located in the middle of the Pacific Ocean.

Concerned communities around the world, from Amsterdam to San Francisco, now require businesses to charge extra for plastic shopping bags or even ban them entirely, encouraging customers to bring their own reusable bags. Take action through inaction, by reducing the amount of plastic bags you acquire in the first place. Refuse plastic bags when offered, and stash canvas totes in your car, bicycle basket, and on doorknobs around your house to remind you to bring them along whenever you head to the store.

Bottled water presents another important opportunity to reduce, reuse, and recycle—again in that order of importance. Moving heavy water from place to place sucks up a lot of fossil fuel energy, and the plastic bottles, while recyclable, often get trashed. One year's worth of plastic bottles, manufactured solely to hold water, uses up 1.5 million barrels of oil. Save money and the planet by purchasing a water filtration system for your home and use it to fill a reusable, stainless steel water bottle so you can hydrate on the go. And don't forget a travel mug for coffee, tea, and soups as well.

Finally, avoid foodstuffs wrapped in unnecessary plastic (like individually wrapped cheese slices), in favor of unpackaged products (i.e., whole or bulk foods), or those contained in glass bottles, cans, or paper.

Unit pricing
Look on grocery shelves for a sticker listing a product's unit price, which reveals the price per pound, quart, or fluid ounce of an item and thus allows you to easily compare prices by weight, no matter what the brand or package size. For example, if coffee brand A comes in a 12-ounce package, and brand B comes in an 18-ounce package, unit pricing will allow you to compare the cost per pound of each at a glance. Unit prices will also allow you to quickly assess the savings whenever you're buying a larger package (sometimes called the "family size") of the exact same item—a strategy that has environmental benefits as well.

PLU codes
These pesky stickers, attached to fruits and vegetables, contain some valuable information for those who know how to decipher them. Four-digit "Product Look-Up" codes denote conventional produce, while a five-digit code, beginning with the number 8, means that the produce in question has been genetically modified. A five-digit code beginning with a 9 means the fruit or vegetable is organic. Gala apples, for example, are PLU #4135. When organically grown, their number is 94135, and if they were genetically modified, that number would be 84135.

Visiting the farmers market
Patronizing that paragon of sustainable shopping—the local farmers market—brings you closer to your community, enables families to stay on their land, and helps conserve open space, in addition to providing you with the freshest, tastiest food. With the help of the Local Harvest Web site, locating markets is easy. Most large cities have a market somewhere every day of the week, and there has been a renaissance in recent years, with more than 4,300 markets operating in the United States today. If your town doesn't have a market, consider

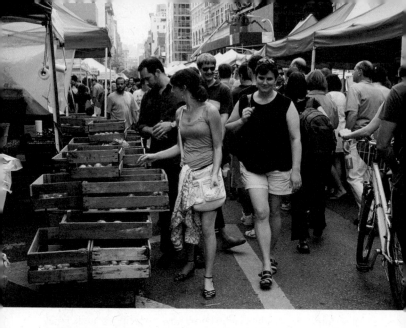

contacting local farmers and organizing with city council members to establish one.

When you visit the market, bring canvas totebags and even a cooler, which will help keep your greens from wilting on the way home, as well as help preserve the freshness of eggs and dairy products. Plan on spending cash (or food stamps), since most vendors aren't equipped to process credit cards, and know that exact change, a "please" and a "thank you," plus a friendly smile are greatly appreciated! Hitting the market in the morning is going to ensure you get popular items, and passing by before closing time will occasionally net you some deals. Writing a list is important, but be flexible, since what's recently harvested and fresh can change from week to week, and you want to be open to surprises. Basing a meal around the bounty of the market can be an extremely fun and challenging exercise, inspiring you to try new recipes for the first time.

Community-supported agriculture

Community-supported agriculture (CSA) has also seen increased interest as the number of educated, concerned consumers grows. Participating in a CSA means you'll receive a weekly delivery of locally grown produce direct from the farm (some CSAs have options for eggs, bread, honey, dairy, fruit, and meat) in exchange for preseason "seed money." The foods that arrive in your weekly basket may not be familiar to you, so ask your farmer for recipes or a newsletter, if the CSA has one. As more people become interested in eating locally, CSAs have begun expanding beyond seasonal shares (spring to fall) and offering year-round packages. Almost all CSA farms are organic, but some choose to forgo the government's expensive certification process, trusting instead that members understand their food will be grown with concern for the environment. Costs vary from farm to farm, and sometimes you may be asked to contribute hours of work as a part of your share. Directly sharing the risks and rewards of farming will bring you into a close relationship with your producer, which in turn helps strengthen the local economy and regional food supply.

Cooking at home

Home-cooked meals cost far less than visiting restaurants, ordering takeout, or even microwaving some prepackaged, "heat 'n' eat" convenience foods, particularly when you consider the value for your money and the environmental impact. Whatever your level of experience, you can prepare simple meals, and, with practice, novice cooks quickly become amazed at how creative and fulfilling cooking can be, while simultaneously developing enthusiasm for healthful, authentic cuisine.

Get your family or friends involved in the kitchen, crank up the tunes, and transform this "chore" into quality time, with a delicious, nutritious, economical, and ecologically friendly feast as your reward. Start simply, with familiar foods like pastas, and easy recipes for mashed potatoes, roasted veggies, or warming soups and casseroles. Also,

ALTERNATIVE MARKETS

Food co-op. Cooperative stores are owned by their members, and they originated as a way for health-conscious food rebels to consolidate their purchasing power. These smaller stores carry more local, organic produce and environmentally friendly products than the supermarket, plus specialty items for vegans and those with food allergies. True co-ops also offer discounts to members, usually in exchange for "sweat equity"—i.e., a few hours of work per week.

Health-food store. Most retail outlets specializing in "health" foods focus on vitamins and protein powders, but many also stock hard-to-find organic products and specialty items.

Farmers market. There's probably no "greener" way to buy your produce than direct from the farmer at a local market. Check localharvest.com to find one near you, and see the section on shopping for more information on this most appealing way to reconnect with the food chain.

Community-supported agriculture. Community-supported agriculture, or CSA, occurs when consumers invest in a farm, buying a "share" in return for a box of seasonal produce that they receive each week during the growing season or, increasingly, year-round. See the previous section on shopping for more information.

Online. Wild salmon, fairly traded dried fruit, coffee, and nuts, plus frozen grass-fed, organic beef, chicken, game, or exotics like buffalo and ostrich, as well as items such as raw nut butters and milks, hemp foods, and interesting ethnic foods can all be ordered online. See the "Resources" section at the back of the book for more on ordering online.

plan to cook more than you need for any given meal, and save the leftovers for lunch the next day. On the weekends, prepare a few extra meals to sustain you during the busy work week.

Grow your own

The freshest, most local, and most affordable produce in the world could literally come from your own backyard, deck, or patio. Starting a garden, even a small one, gives you an opportunity to grow your own organic vegetables, fruits, and herbs at a fraction of the cost of supermarket prices, while eliminating the need for shipping and storage that contributes to the industrial food system's large "carbon footprint." Best of all, nothing tastes better—or makes you feel more connected to your meal and Mother Nature—than enjoying a source of nourishment that started out as a small seed in your own hands.

Even apartment dwellers can grow plants in window boxes, on fire escapes, or up on the roof. Start with easy-to-grow and versatile plants like basil, garlic, parsley, tomatoes, cucumbers, strawberries, lettuces, and greens like arugula, chard, and kale. Don't forget to include beautiful varieties of edible flowers, like nasturtiums and violas.

Community gardens offer another excellent opportunity for those without much space to get growing. You can find one nearby at communitygarden.org.

Composting

Eliminate food scraps from your household garbage, keep biodegradable waste out of our overused landfills, and provide superrich soil for your backyard garden at the same time by constructing and maintaining your own compost pile. Check out *Composting: An Easy Household Guide* by Nicky Scott for more information.

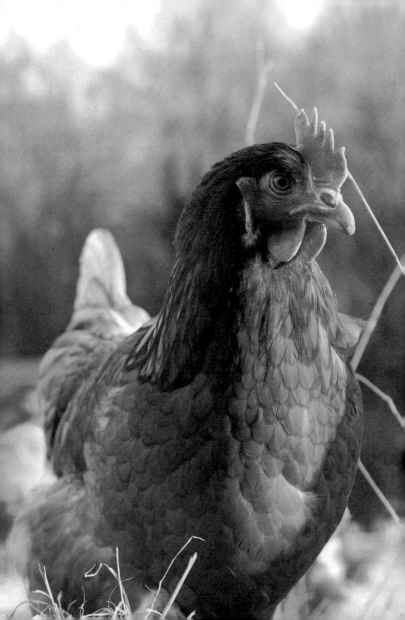

Chapter 1

BEEF, PORK, AND POULTRY

Hunting animals for food marked a pivotal step in human evolution, one that required courage, teamwork, strategy, and determination. After a successful outing, ancient hunters would share their spoils with all the members of their tribe, tightening the bonds of society and forming the basis for the ceremonial meals we still enjoy today. But keep in mind that for our distant ancestors a successful kill proved relatively rare, and so they still relied on gathering plant foods more than hunting game for day-to-day survival.

Over time, the domestication of food animals and the widespread establishment of agriculture somewhat insulated humankind from the harshest laws of nature. Fast-forward many thousands of years to the postindustrial era, and this insulation has grown so complete that we see a great rift in people's understanding of exactly how food animals live and die. With consumers so far removed from the unpleasantness of "the kill," many of us unquestioningly take for granted the packaged, precut meats found in refrigerated supermarket cases and enjoy this abundance of flesh in blissful ignorance.

Ask around and you'll find that few people want to know the dirty details of how today's factory farms raise cattle, hogs, and chickens. Even fewer can stalk, capture, kill, butcher, and prepare a wild animal for dinner. This lack of primary knowledge has led to a distortion of our role as predators and a corruption of our rightful place in the food chain. Instead of balancing our diets to suit the natural world, we've overwhelmed it, creating an imbalance that's starkly evident in how our culture deals with meat.

Most Americans eat meat every day, many at every meal, and this overconsumption leads to negative consequences for both the environment and our health. By choosing to eat less meat, and consuming meat that has been properly raised, you can return proper balance to your own diet, foster better health, and help create a cleaner environment along the way.

What's Wrong with Factory Farms?

Meat production, as realized in confined animal feeding operations (CAFOs), a.k.a. "factory farms" — in other words, the conventional method of bringing meat to market in the United States—involves shipping young steers, hogs, chickens, and other livestock to feedlots to be fattened and slaughtered. These "animal cities" concentrate huge populations in cramped stalls or cages, where they're unable to escape their own filth or engage in natural, innate behaviors such as grazing, rooting, or roosting—crowding that inevitably leads to problems with animal health and waste management.

Most of the corn and soybeans grown in America are used for animal feed at CAFOs. The cultivation of these genetically modified crops requires enormous amounts of energy to power heavy farm machinery, plus large inputs of synthetic fertilizers, as well as chemical pest and weed controls, all of them petroleum-based, and all of which run off directly into our surface or ground waters, with disastrous results. In fact, there's no method of food production more ecologically damaging than modern CAFOs, which, owing to their intense feeding needs, account for 60 percent of all pesticide use and 70 percent of all water use.

With a yield of 1 calorie of red meat for every 78 calories of fossil fuel, consuming burgers and steaks also contributes mightily to climate change—and that's before you even consider the methane emissions from the cattle farts! Also, CAFOs concentrate manure into giant pools that overwhelm the ecosystems around them, turning an invaluable fertilizer into a waste-management problem. When this toxic animal waste overflows into waterways, it kills fish by the thousands and causes tremendous pollution.

Unfortunately, for too many of us, these steep, unjustifiable costs of factory farming aren't figured into the price of "cheap" meat.

Health: Hormones and Antibiotics in Meat

In addition to its environmental degradation, the health risks associated with conventionally produced meat can be dire indeed. There's no knowing what sort of diet your factory-farmed burger, bacon, or chicken "nugget" was raised on (by the way, what part of the chicken exactly does the "nugget" come from?), nor the quantity of pharmaceuticals pumped into the animal while it was alive. CAFOs produce meat cheaply because they fatten livestock quickly, feeding them high-calorie grain and prohibiting much exercise.

For the purpose of promoting the growth of broiler chickens and improving the color of their meat, the FDA approves the use of arsenic to supplement chicken feed. In the form of roxarsone, this additive breaks down in the bird's body to more harmful, carcinogenic compounds called arsenite and arsenate. Certified organic chicken is arsenic-free, which not only preserves your health, but also prevents chicken manure laced with arsenic from being applied to cropland as fertilizer.

Beef cattle and dairy cows are also fed all manner of industrial by-products, from chicken manure to stale bubblegum. Since these ruminant animals evolved to eat grass, this unnatural diet of grain and garbage causes cattle to develop bloat. Once sickened, livestock constantly require low doses of antibiotics to continue the fattening operation. The subtherapeutic use of these medications to produce cheap meat, eggs, and milk creates new bacterial strains that are resistant to antibiotics, exposing humans to nasty, multidrug-resistant infections that are more difficult, if not impossible, to control. Growth hormones are also given to animals to increase their size, affecting human health in as yet unknown ways.

Take action to prevent the massive pollution, cruelty, and disease that represent the side effects of industrial meat production. Protest factory farming, boycott its products, eat less meat overall, and use the money you save to support sustainable, natural, healthy farming methods.

Off the Meaten Path

Add diversity to your diet and avoid factory farming by seeking out locally sourced meats from small-scale farms. Animals such as bison, lamb, duck, rabbit, and ostrich often offer a more viable alternative to CAFO products. Many small livestock concerns also raise heritage breeds, such as Devon cattle or Shetland sheep—domesticated species that have become increasingly rare. Preserving heritage breeds protects genetic diversity, and many of these animals have unique disease resistance or other special adaptations.

From the pasture to the plate

Organic and grass-fed beef, bison, pork, and poultry offer a healthier, more socially responsible alternative to factory-farmed meats, eliminating many of the harmful side effects caused by CAFOs. Animals raised outdoors and fed natural grass live the way nature intended, and their pastures utilize the energy of the sun efficiently, growing grass abundantly without the copious chemical inputs required by the crops of corn and soy grown to service factory feedlots.

The native grasses grown to feed naturally pastured cattle also sequester massive amounts of carbon dioxide underground in their giant root systems—more than enough to offset the methane gas (from flatulence) naturally released by livestock. This means that, unlike herds raised in CAFOs, pasture-raised cattle don't contribute to global warming. The native grasses' intertwining root systems also virtually eliminate the erosion of precious topsoil, which is not always the case in cultivated, tilled fields.

Farmers who raise pastured livestock take pride in managing their land with an eye to the future. Many employ "conservation" or "rotational grazing" methods, moving their animals from parcel to parcel

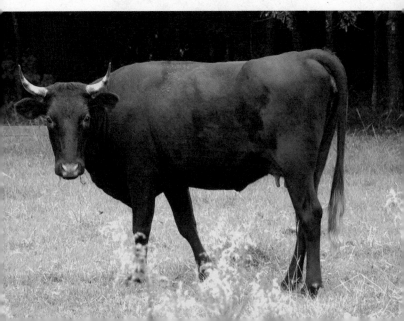

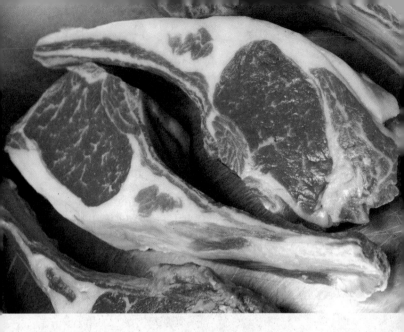

as each is grazed, a process designed to mimic the impact of native grazers like deer or elk. Well-managed pasture has excellent soil stability, more earthworms, and better wildlife habitat than a field of row crops. In this cyclical, sustainable system, cattle spread manure that nourishes the soil, which provides lush grass, which later feeds the same cattle. Compare this balanced, natural system to the manure lagoons maintained by CAFOs, and you'll see that raising livestock on pasture is a commonsense solution to a number of industrial problems. Also, grass-fed cattle eat their natural diet, so they do not sicken and therefore do not require nonstop antibiotic treatment.

Health benefits of grass-fed meat
It takes longer to fatten grass-fed steers, which makes their meat more expensive, but you'll find the nutritional benefits and finer taste justify the expense, particularly once you resolve to eat less—and better—meat.

Gaining in popularity nationwide, bison burgers have shown up on trendy restaurant menus, and the meat is available frozen in many stores or online. Native to prairie grasslands, the comeback of the almost-obliterated bison should be celebrated and supported as an alternative to CAFO steers. Fed on grass, bison meat has 70 to 90 percent less saturated fat, 50 percent less cholesterol, and is higher in protein, iron, omega-3 fatty acid, and amino acids.

The diet that livestock eat is undeniably linked to the end quality of their meat. Grass has twenty times more vitamin E than soy or corn, so cattle fed grass absorb much more vitamin E into their flesh. Pastured meat is also rich in conjugated linoleic acid (CLA), a cancer-fighting "good fat," as well as omega-3s. (CAFO meat, fed on grain and garbage, does not have these nutritional benefits.) While "good fats" are abundant, the total content of saturated fat in grass-fed beef is much lower than the conventional product, making moderate consumption of grass-fed meat a suitable choice for omnivores working to lose weight. The nutritional benefits of pastured meat and eggs are further detailed at Jo Robinson's excellent Eat Wild Web site (listed in the "Resources" section), along with many resources for locating suppliers near you.

Hunting
Despite its "barbaric" reputation, hunting can actually represent a sustainable and socially responsible way to enjoy meat. As a group, hunters also help ensure the preservation of wild lands while maintaining a realistic perspective on our place in the food chain. Imagine a scheme that would seek to address exploding deer populations by allowing local, wild venison to be processed and sold at farmers markets. While the USDA currently lacks the regulatory framework to adapt ingenious, appropriate ideas such as this to help solve our burgeoning ecological problems, local activists can work to make partnerships between hunters, environmentalists, and foodies.

From the Nest

Eggs may be one of nature's most nutritionally balanced foods, but conventional methods of production involve raising animals in extremely inhumane conditions. In addition to the resulting environmental degradation, conventional eggs laid by crowded, stressed hens lead to an increased risk of salmonella poisoning, so if you're fond of runny yolks or need to use raw eggs for a recipe, always source your eggs from organic farmers with small, free-ranging flocks.

In a traditional farmyard setting, chickens eat insects, grass, and seeds. Pastured poultry produce eggs with less cholesterol and saturated fat, and more vitamins A, E, and B12, and omega-3s. Look for pasture-raised eggs at farmers markets, purchase cage-free, organic eggs at the grocery store, or even look into raising your own backyard flock. Chickens are relatively easy to keep, and they eat kitchen scraps as well as keep your lawn free of grubs. Check the regulations where you live to find out if backyard flocks are permitted, but avoid raising a noisy rooster in densely populated places. Sharing eggs with neighbors is a great way to build community and awareness of local food.

Becoming Vegetarian (or Flexitarian)

Caring for the future of our planet means no longer applying industrial logic to meat production. Sustainable, pasture-raised meat and eggs may be more expensive, but that's only because they reflect the true, unsubsidized costs of raising healthy animals. The economic forces that make factory-farmed meat so cheap are also what lead to cruelty, negative health conditions, and environmental damage. Therefore, one of the best actions you can take to lessen environmental degradation and improve your health is to buy smaller amounts of higher-quality organic or grass-fed meat, and use it in recipes that heighten these unique, rich flavors.

Challenge the notion that large portions of meat must occupy the center of the plate, with the rest of a meal revolving around it. This isn't how most of the world eats. Until recently, beef was an expensive luxury, as evidenced by older recipes for stews and casseroles that stretched each bit of meat as much as possible.

But what about eliminating meat from your diet entirely?

Vegetarianism can be intimidating even for people consciously considering ethical choices. Rather than expecting yourself, much less everyone in America, to immediately boycott all meats, it may be more realistic to work toward incremental change. Truly, there is no right diet for everyone, so, regardless of the environmental benefits, bullying people into adopting a meat-free lifestyle can prove counterproductive. Instead, vegetarians and vegans can lead by example, enticing friends and family with delicious meat-free meals, shared with a positive attitude, while encouraging any moves in the right direction.

Going vegetarian is also an effective way to trim your grocery budget. The savings earned by abstaining from meat can easily finance purchases of organic produce. If you'd still like to indulge occasionally, choose organic chicken over industrial beef—the price should be about equal.

No matter which course you decide to pursue, no one who eats meat should do so while remaining ignorant of the consequences one's lifestyle has for the environment and its negative effects on one's health. If you'd like to do your part for the environment, but can't commit to total meat abstinence, consider joining the growing ranks of the flexitarians. To become one, simply reduce your frequency of carnivorous meals. If you currently eat meat three times a day, decide to have it only once. If you currently eat meat once a day, cut down to two or three servings per week. Gradually increase the number of

WHAT TO LOOK FOR ON MEAT AND EGG LABELS

Grass-Fed or Pastured. *Cattle, hogs, goats, chickens, or sheep that eat grass and roots from spring to fall and hay during the winter can be called grass-fed or pastured. The advantages to growing meat this way are many, including preservation of rural landscapes, and the elimination of pesticide pollution and topsoil erosion. Grass-fed meat is also much healthier for humans to consume, and usually does not contain antibiotics or hormones. Please note, occasionally livestock raised indoors are labeled as "Grass-fed," while the term "Pastured" indicates the animal was raised outdoors in a traditional manner. The phrase "Grain-supplemented" indicates that grain was added to the animal's diet, but in a limited way that doesn't cause sickness.*

Certified Humane. *Produced according to the rigorous standards of Humane Farm Animal Care, a nonprofit aligned with the Royal Society for the Prevention of Cruelty to Animals, meat with the "Certified Humane" logo was treated as well as can be expected from birth to slaughter. The criteria developed by HFAC addresses the animal's health, management, and environment, and can be applied to beef cattle, dairy cows, poultry chickens, egg-laying hens, and goats.*

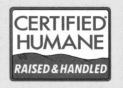

Organic. *Meat with a USDA "Certified Organic" seal on it was raised on organic feed, and contains zero antibiotics or growth hormones. Organic meat was not raised "grass-fed" unless the label specifically says so, despite any bucolic illustrations and logo designs on the packaging showing happy animals on an endless pasture.*

No Animal By-Products. *This label means that livestock were not fed the offal of any other animal. The attention-grabbing label "No Animal Cannibalism" means the same thing. In 2003, after the outbreak of mad cow disease, the USDA banned feedlots in the United States from using tissues from the nervous systems of sheep, goats, or cattle to feed to other ani-*

mals, but many other animal by-products still find their way into factory farm feed.

Free-Range. Free-range animals live outside of a cage and are allowed to wander and engage in natural behaviors. The USDA regulates the use of the term when applied to poultry that's raised to be eaten, mandating that birds have access to the outdoors for a set amount of time each day. The term is not regulated when applied to egg-laying hens or cattle, whether raised for meat or dairy.

Cage-Free. Outrage at the use of battery cages, which confine birds in a very small space, stacked on top of each other, has led many consumers to seek out cage-free eggs.

Cage-free isn't cruelty-free, but birds are given more space, can stretch their wings, walk around, and dust-bathe.

Nitrate- or Nitrite-Free. Synthetic nitrates and nitrites are found in all commercially cured meat, and they have been connected to increased risks of certain cancers, as well as to triggering asthma attacks or causing headaches or dizziness. Any naturally "cured" meat product—such as bacon, ham, sausage, salami, pepperoni, jerky, or lunchmeat—produced without synthetic nitrates and nitrites earns the label "Nitrate/Nitrite Free." These products use nitrates and nitrites from natural sources to prevent spoilage or bacterial contamination.

Natural. The label "Natural" has been so overused and underregulated that it means basically nothing. According to the Food Safety and Inspection Service (FSIS), "natural" should indicate a minimally processed product containing no artificial flavors, colors, or preservatives. Plus, any other company claims on the package should be truthful, such as "No Antibiotics" or "All-Vegetable Diet," but no inspections enforce the use of the label "natural," or any other uncertified company claims. The USDA allows packers to use words like "fresh" and "natural" on any unfrozen meat that has been unaltered before slaughter. Unfortunately, the USDA does not consider the use of hormones or antibiotics as an applicable "alteration."

"vegetarian days" in your week, while allowing yourself "cultural exceptions" for holidays, dinner parties, or vacations.

Flexitarians can also choose a new dietary philosophy that lets meat be an accompaniment, and moves plant foods to the center of the plate. (This approach is central to *The Ethical Gourmet*—see the "Resources" section—a groundbreaking cookbook with tons of recipes.)

Several strategies exist that allow you to reduce the amount of meat you consume without feeling deprived. Eating meat along with complex carbohydrates—a technique known as "protein sparing"—requires a smaller portion of meat to fulfill your daily requirement of essential amino acids and achieve a satiated feeling. Plenty of protein to maintain good health can be found in beans, nuts, and grains. If you successfully quit meat, yet find yourself craving it very often or thinking about it constantly, cease your obsessing and heed your body's message. Allow for a few "nonvegetarian" days where you indulge in a grass-fed burger.

If you kick the carnivorous habit completely, then congratulate yourself! Use your savings from the old "beef budget" to reward yourself with an excellent cookbook, a sharp chef's knife, or new cutting board. Your body and mind will also reward you, with years of good health and a clean conscience.

Meat Substitutes

Imitation "meat" products, called soy analogs, include fake foods like Boca "burgers," Tofu Pups, and Chik'n patties. Many tasty homemade vegetarian chili recipes contain texturized vegetable protein (TVP) "beef" crumbles. You can even find high-end restaurants that serve elaborate "mock meat" entrees.

WHERE'S THE BEEF?

The following is a crash course on common meaty stand-ins. These are not soy analogs; they're minimally processed ingredients that can always have a place on your plate.

Tofu. *Soybean curd is useful in a variety of traditional Asian dishes, but not when it's pretending to be a hot dog or turkey. Tofu is bland, making it a perfect base for soaking up flavors and spices. Different textures include silken, soft, firm, and extra-firm; use the first two for smoothies or dips, and the last two for stir-fries or baking.*

Tempeh. *Whole soybeans inoculated with a mold; the resulting tempeh cake is bound together by a ferment. Tempeh has a nutty flavor, and is excellent in a variety of recipes.*

Seiten. *Protein-rich wheat gluten that remains after the rest of the flour is washed away. Chewy and absorbent, seiten is easy to make at home and can also be found in specialty stores.*

While these choices are ethically superior to CAFO meat in many ways, and have helped many people more easily transition to a meat-free lifestyle, soy analogs remain heavily processed foods, sometimes containing many preservatives, artificial flavors, and colorings. Also, the extensive refining, packaging, and refrigeration that soy-analog products require isn't healthy or sustainable. In contrast, excellent veggie burgers made with rice and lentils are both satisfying and sustainable.

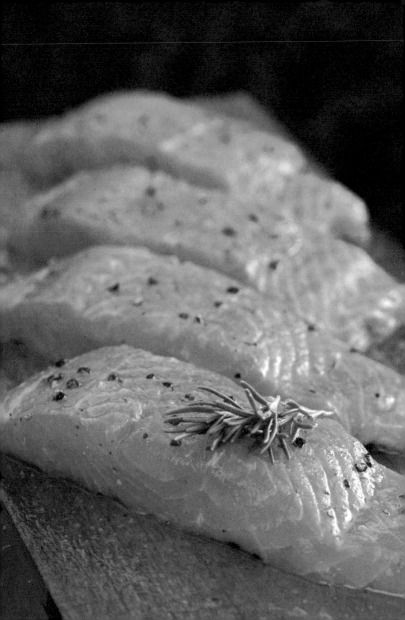

Chapter 2

FISH AND SEAFOOD

For most Americans, fish and seafood represent the only wild foods found in their diet. Consequently, mindful consumers shopping for sustainable selections will encounter a series of complicated considerations that go way beyond price per pound and freshness. Venture over to the fish and seafood counter in your supermarket, or even visit a local fish merchant or seafood restaurant, and your purchasing decisions will have dramatic effects on both your own health and the well-being of the planet.

Making informed decisions starts with learning all you can about different species, including their biology and reproductive cycles, geographic range, and place in the oceanic food chain—not to mention where they came from, whether they were fresh or frozen, "wild caught" or "farm raised." Trying to be ethical, economical, and epicurean all at once can be overwhelming enough to make you shrug and reach for the canned tuna, but take heart: We'll cover the basics here, and groups like the Marine Stewardship Council (msc.org) can provide you with more detailed information on tasty, affordable, guilt-free fish and seafood options.

General Fish Tips

When shopping for fish at market, always select the freshest possible. Fresh fish shouldn't have an odor of excessive "fishiness," or ammonia.

The flesh should be firm, and bounce back when pressed by a finger. Fish on display should always be on ice, but not buried in ice, and the ice shouldn't be melted.

Fresh fish is preferable to frozen, and while canned fish is convenient, the canning process is very energy-intensive. By weight, canned fish may also be more expensive than fresh fish. Smoked and dried fish are preferable to canned, and there are excellent varieties of tuna "jerky" on the market today.

Environmental Issues: Overfishing, Loss of Habitat, and Species Depletion

Despite the vastness of the oceans, the fish and seafood harvested from them are far from limitless. Alarmed by the worldwide collapse of fisheries, environmental activists estimate that 90 percent of the large, predatory species in the sea now teeter on the brink of extinction. And the commercial fishing industry's shortsighted, industrial perspective on utilizing oceanic ecosystems means that vessels from different countries continue to compete for the same fish in the same areas, many using increasingly destructive and sophisticated technology to pull greater harvests from an ever-diminishing supply.

Instead of partnering with environmental groups to implement strict regulations necessary to protect and conserve fish species, thus preserving this precious food supply (not to mention the fishing trade itself) for future generations, most commercial fishing operations instead focus solely on harvesting as many fish as possible from the oceans before they're all gone. Meanwhile, a lack of political action at all levels of government means that, despite the environmental risks, you will continue to find increasingly rare species in markets and on menus, including bluefin tuna, red snapper, grouper, orange roughy, and Chilean sea bass (also called Patagonian toothfish). We must all act now to reverse this dangerous trend, or else, one day, these and many other species will disappear, never to be seen or eaten again.

The consumer movement for dolphin-safe tuna provides a successful model that can be replicated to protect other at-risk species. We all deserve sustainable oceans, and safe, healthy fish and seafood.

Fish Farms: Good or Bad?

Farm-raised fish and seafood presents a dilemma for eco-conscious consumers. When it comes to buying the products of aquaculture, the environmental impact of your purchase could be benign or could be disastrous, depending on the species of fish, the location of the farm, and the methods employed in raising, harvesting, and transporting your next dinner. And so it's important to educate yourself before things get fishy.

For instance, aquaculture farms producing Atlantic salmon greatly contribute to ocean pollution, and potentially spread diseases from farmed fish to endangered wild ones. Crowded into offshore pens, these farmed fish are fed antibiotics in order to control disease. Also, since salmon are carnivorous, they need to eat many smaller fish. When farm-raised, this means ground-up fish pellets, which give a gray coloration to the flesh (as opposed to wild salmon, which dine on crustaceans, giving their flesh its characteristic pink color). Since gray salmon isn't very appetizing, farmed fish get fed a synthetic pigment produced by a pharmaceutical firm to replicate the natural color of wild salmon.

Also, to promote faster growth, farmed salmon are genetically altered, which is good for the industry, because the fish will not need to eat so many food pellets, but presents significant problems when these GM fish escape into the ecosystem and compete against wild

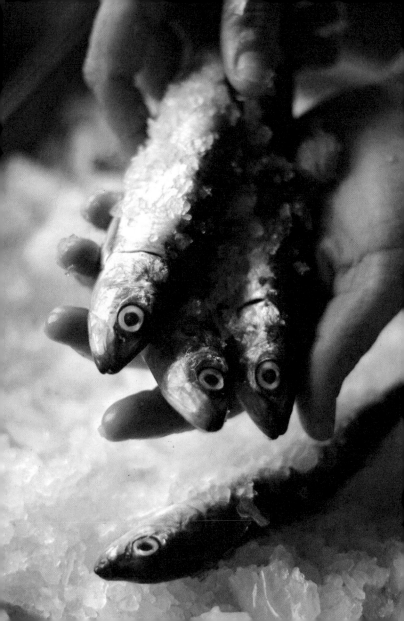

salmon for food and mates. Together, all these drawbacks make genetically modified, antibiotic-laden, artificially colored farmed salmon a poor substitute for real, wild salmon, which can be obtained from responsibly managed fisheries in Alaska, or ordered online from services such as Vital Choice.

On the other hand, successful, sustainable fish farms do exist, ones that build on the symbiotic relationships between fish and plants found in nature. For instance, farmers in the Mississippi River and in Asian rice paddies raise catfish, tilapia, and crawfish in aquaculture systems that have beneficial or neutral effects on the ecosystem. Shellfish perform a vital service in filtering water from estuaries and wetlands, and so farmed mussels, oysters, and clams are also an ecologically sound purchase. Other farmed species that can be recommended include Arctic char, sturgeon, barramundi, striped bass, rainbow trout, and bay scallops. In general, fish farmed in rivers or inland ponds are preferable to fish farmed in the ocean, and choosing fish farmed in the United States also encourages local economies and reduces the energy used in bringing them to market.

Health Risks: Mercury and PCBs

A toxic by-product of coal-burning power plants, methyl mercury spreads through watersheds to the ocean, where it accumulates in the bodies of fish. Mercury harms humans by disrupting the neurological system, and is extremely dangerous for pregnant women and young children, whose still-developing brains and nervous systems are much more vulnerable to impairment. This means women of childbearing age and children under twelve should limit their intake of fish to no more than one small serving per week. The rest of us can safely consume a little more, but make no mistake, the dangers posed by heavy metals and chemicals have tainted most large fish.

LABELS TO LOOK FOR ON FISH

Country of Origin. In 2005, laws mandating country-of-origin labeling (COOL) came into effect that require seafood counters to inform consumers if, for example, the catfish on display is from Vietnam or the United States. This information is of great help to consumers, provided they know that farmed salmon from Chile is environmentally suspect, while wild salmon from Alaska is managed well.

Farmed. All farmed fish must be labeled as such. You can assume that unless labeled otherwise, all salmon and shrimp are farmed. Aquaculture isn't all bad: just stay away from Atlantic salmon and stick to U.S.-farmed catfish, tilapia, Arctic char, sturgeon, barramundi, striped bass, rainbow trout, bay scallops, clams, mussels, or oysters.

Marine Stewardship Council. This nonprofit organization certifies responsible fisheries using sustainable management methods that minimize by-catch and industry pollution, maintain breeding populations to replacement levels, and take a long-term approach to preserving healthy ecosystems, and thus, the future of the fishery. Find more info at www.msc.org

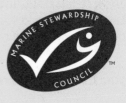

Organic. The USDA maintains no official standards for organic seafood. Some fish and seafood is marketed as organic, however, because, in lieu of a set of government-regulated rules, private certifying agencies have

Fish at the upper end of the food chain eat many smaller fish, which means greater concentrations of mercury and other pollutants, such as PCBs and dioxins, build up in their bodies. Consequently, sharks, swordfish, marlin, tilefish, and giant tunas, such as bluefins, harbor gone ahead and adapted livestock standards to seafood, in order to service companies who want recognition for their efforts toward sustainability. It's worth Googling the company and certifying agency before paying the higher price.

Seafood Safe. Each year, seafood distributor EcoFish collects seven samples of the frozen fish it distributes, and has them tested for mercury and PCBs. Based on their findings, they print a number in red on their packaging label to indicate the amount of 4-ounce servings of this type of fish it's safe for a 140-pound woman of childbearing age to consume in one month. Serving suggestions for other adults and children can be found on their Web site at www.seafoodsafe.com

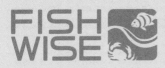

FishWise. Developed by Sustainable Fishery Advocates, a nonprofit organization that works closely with the Monterey Bay Aquarium, color-coded FishWise labels are applied by the retailer, and alert consumers to potential problems with a fishery. Green indicates that the fish is caught using nondestructive methods, and the population is healthy; red indicates that the population is in dangerous decline; and yellow designates a middle ground between the two. More information is available at www.fishwise.org

the most toxins. (Giant tunas and some shark species are also in the most danger of extinction.) Meanwhile, "chunk light" canned tunas are smaller, cheaper, and contain three times less mercury than albacore tuna.

Carnivorous farmed fish, like Atlantic salmon, are generally higher in harmful pollutants than their wild equivalents. These toxins have been found to increase cancer risk in women and girls who consistently consume farmed salmon. Chemicals accumulate in fatty tissues, which means you can lessen some of your toxin exposure by avoiding fatty fish skins.

Get Your Omega-3s

Omega-3 fatty acids—essential for optimal brain and nervous system function as well as preventing a number of diseases and mood disorders—are the primary health benefit humans derive from fish. Unfortunately, the fish richest in omega-3s—fatty fish from cold waters, such as salmon and bluefish—also happen to be the most polluted, endangered, and environmentally suspect. Better fish sources for omega-3s include small fish such as anchovies and sardines, but omega-3s are also available from specially fortified eggs (laid by hens fed diets rich in omega-3s), grass-fed meats and eggs, flax seeds, hemp seeds, walnuts, or fish-oil supplements that have been purified to remove mercury.

Fish for the Future

It's tough to be an environmentally conscious sushi lover these days, but certain sustainable choices remain available. Remember that, in the United States, the vast majority of fish and seafood is eaten in restaurants, where responsible chefs have an opportunity to make a real difference for the future of the world's oceans. If you ever see a menu featuring an endangered fish like Chilean sea bass, mention it to your server or the manager. Any well-run restaurant will be responsive to respectfully submitted customer concerns.

When dining out or at home, reject predatory fish like sharks, farmed salmon, and giant tunas (ahi, bluefin, yellowfin), and rare fish like grouper, red snapper, orange roughy, Chilean sea bass, Atlantic cod, monkfish, flounder, and haddock in favor of smaller, fast-growing fish, such as anchovies, sardines, mackerel, smelt, and herring. Mahi-mahi, also called dorado, is a large, tasty fish that reproduces quickly, and so remains a sustainable choice for the time being. Choose wild Alaskan pollock or salmon, Pacific halibut, striped sea bass, or any of the farmed options recommended above (pg 19). For fans of crustaceans, Dungeness crabs and stone crabs get the "eco-OK," along with spiny lobsters from the United States. For more detailed information on a wide variety of farm-raised and wild fish and seafood, consult the Monterey Bay Aquarium's Web site at www.montereybay aquarium.org.

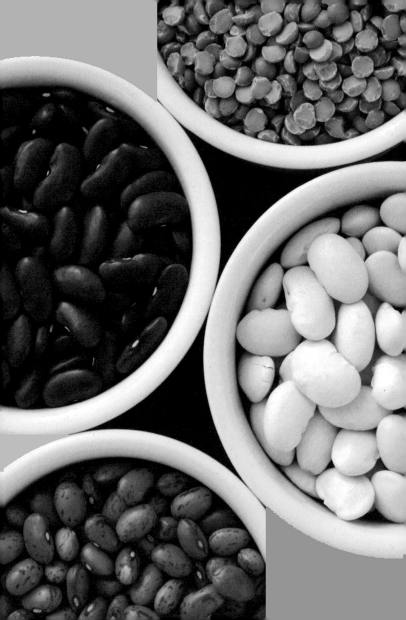

Chapter 3

GRAINS, BEANS, AND NUTS

Grains

When most Americans think of grain, "amber waves of grain" immediately comes to mind, as in the massive fields of wheat that make up the country's "breadbasket." *God Bless America*, however, fails to include a line about dousing those amber waves in agrochemicals, including toxic fertilizers and pesticides. Buying organic flour eliminates these harmful processes, protecting both your health and the environment.

Also, while it's nice to have a palate that's "refined," the opposite holds true when it comes to your wheat. The process of refining grains removes essential nutrients found in the plant, and while a few of these nutrients can be added back in an industrial process known as fortification, still, over time, a diet too high in refined flours and processed foods will have detrimental effects on health.

Meanwhile, whole grains contain all three parts of the plant—hull, endosperm, and germ—providing the kind of balanced nourishment our bodies have evolved to digest properly. The hull is the grain's fibrous outer covering, and contains much of the plant's nutrients. The germ is the fatty, oilier part, often removed in the refining process because it can go rancid and reduce shelf life. The endosperm is the starchy part, which refining preserves, while discarding the hull (also known as bran) and germ.

Whole grains are chewy, textured, and can take a long time to cook. Grinding, or "milling," whole grains makes them easier to prepare and digest without sacrificing taste or nutritional balance. Milled grains first become grits or "cracked grains," the most familiar being corn grits and steel-cut oats. Further milling creates "flakes," such as oatmeal. It's only in the last milling step, when grains are ground into flour, that refining comes into play. By purchasing whole-wheat flour, you can skip this final, detrimental step.

The simplest way to revive a tired weekly menu routine is to learn how to cook a new whole grain and use it in place of an old standard. Replacing refined carbohydrates like white bread and white rice with minimally processed whole grains like barley, oats, and brown rice will ensure you're eating the healthiest and tastiest meals possible, and can also save you money. If you eat a lot of potatoes, switch it up one night and try bulgur (an extremely quick-cooking form of wheat grits) or couscous (not a true grain, but tiny pasta made of semolina flour). Polished barley is similar in appearance and texture to rice, and polenta (corn grits) pairs nicely with many of the sauces and vegetables that accompany pasta.

Also, why pay the packaged-food industry to transform delicious, nutritious ears of farm-fresh corn into a bag of salty, unsatisfying corn chips that are also potentially loaded with other unhealthy food additives?

And finally, consider experimenting with some "ancient" grains that may be new or unfamiliar to modern consumers, such as quinoa, kasha (aka buckwheat), amaranth, and teff. (Quinoa, amaranth and kasha aren't technically grains, but are used similarly, so they fall into this group.) Increasingly, allergies to wheat and gluten are becoming more common. People who suffer from these allergies often tolerate ancient grains like amaranth and spelt. Many exotic rice varieties can also be found in markets, and cooking with basmati, wehani, or wild rice (actually not related to cultivated rice, but the seed of a native wetlands grass) is a way to add new life to stir-fries, pilafs, and other familiar dishes.

As always, look for organic labels on grains, and be sure to avoid white, refined foods, whether breads, rice, or flour, in favor of minimally processed whole grains.

"Less Than Daily" Bread

Lowering your intake of white bread, especially mass-produced, presliced "Wonder"-type bread, will undoubtedly be good for your health. Baked goods made from refined flour—such as white bread, cakes, or muffins—raise your blood sugar quickly, causing your pancreas to work harder secreting more insulin to convert the carbohydrate sugars into a form your cells can assimilate. Whole grains, on the other hand, are assimilated slowly by the body, providing sustained energy.

You can also use the money you save by buying less to buy better, including occasionally splurging on artisanal breads like sourdough, foccacia, and challah, which can effortlessly elevate even the simplest sandwich into a work of art. When shopping for presliced breads, look for organic, whole-grain loaves. Sprouted breads, produced without honey, eggs, or oil, are also excellent for your health, and they have a distinctly toothsome texture that's really tasty when toasted. Reject any bread made with high-fructose corn syrup, which is a telltale sign of junky food. In fact, reject *anything* with the dreaded HFCS!

Finally, instead of throwing out stale artisanal bread products, get thrifty and gourmet at the same time by transforming them into delicious stratas, soups, puddings, or croutons.

Beans

Despite the popular ditty, beans are neither magical nor a fruit, but they do represent a perfect example of a whole plant food that's high in fiber and protein. They're also simple to cook and can be used in diverse recipes gleaned from cultures all around the globe.

Popular bean varieties include cannellini (white), Great Northern, kidney (red), black, adzuki, garbanzos (chickpeas), pinto, soy, lima, fava, and lentils, with more heirloom varieties available all the time! Lentils are especially versatile, cook quickly, and don't need to be soaked before cooking. As with any other type of vegetable, fruit, or grain, use organic varieties of beans whenever you can afford to, especially when choosing canned beans, since organic brands usually contain less salt. Still, any variety of canned beans should be rinsed in a colander before using to remove excess sodium.

Soybeans aren't commonly eaten at the table, since they take a long time to cook and are difficult to digest, except in the form of edamame—fresh, whole, young soybeans that have been steamed and salted and are served in their pods. Otherwise, consume high-protein soybeans in traditional, minimally processed forms such as tofu, tempeh, miso, and in soy sauces—all tasty, healthy ways to enjoy your soy.

Buying dried beans will save you money, but not necessarily time, although there's some debate over whether or not it's necessary for dried beans (other than lentils) to be soaked overnight. A lot depends on the age of your beans; if they're too old, as in over two years, all the soaking in the world may not render them edible. For added convenience, soak and cook a large amount of beans over the weekend, then save unused, prepared beans in the fridge for recipes later in the week. Cooked beans will keep for up to five days.

Going Nuts (and Seeds)

Nuts have been much maligned as being high in fat, but they contain the good kind of fat, as well as being a delicious whole food that provides quick energy. Buy nuts in their shells whenever possible, as this usually means they will be cheaper, and their natural "packaging" prevents them from going rancid too quickly. Either way, all nuts should be stored in the refrigerator or freezer because of their high oil content.

Keeping almonds, hazelnuts, cashews, and peanuts (the latter two are not technically nuts), or whatever nut you enjoy munching on handy provides an easy snacking option that may not seem cheap until you compare it to the costs (financial, health, environmental, and otherwise) of packaged snacks made of processed foods. You can roast or salt nuts easily enough yourself, so avoid buying "salted" varieties or pre-roasted nuts, which, despite their name, have most likely been fried. Also, check the nutritional label for the presence of added sweeteners or salt.

You can support important environmental goals and your own taste buds by choosing Brazil nuts. These large, luxurious nuts grow in the rainforest on trees that can produce for a thousand years, but resist being cultivated. A steady market for Brazil nuts ensures the survival of the wild rainforest, and that those who gather them receive a fair wage. For more information about seeking out fair-trade products, see pg. 55.

For raw foodists (see pg. xviii), much like the "primitive" eaters they emulate, nuts are an indispensable source of protein. Any raw-food diet will rely on seeds, nuts, nut butters, and nut milks—an excellent replacement for dairy. Creamy "milks" made from cashews or almonds can be used in many recipes in place of cream, or even poured on top of your (all-natural) breakfast cereal.

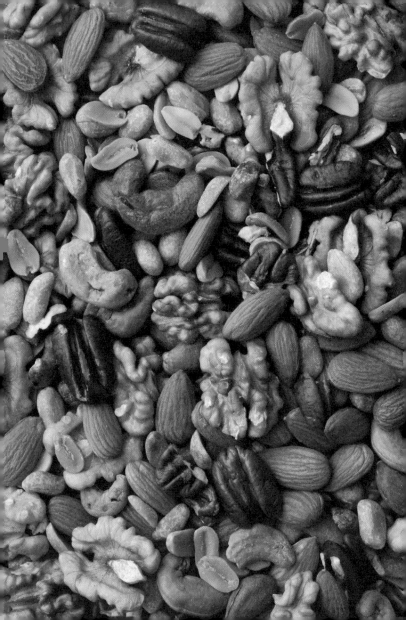

Seeds also make great snacks, and can be integrated into many recipes, baked into breads and muffins, or sprinkled on salads. Seeds from sunflowers and pumpkins, and flax, hemp, and sesame seeds all contain protein, fiber, and essential amino acids; hemp and flax also provide lots of balanced omega-3 and omega-6 fatty acids. Sprouted seeds, like sunflowers or "microgreens," provide a great pick-me-up in the winter when the fresh baby greens of spring remain weeks away. However, avoid eating raw any sprouted legumes, such as alfalfa, mung bean, or chickpea sprouts; these contain natural toxins that are, however, destroyed by cooking, rendering them safe and delicious.

If cooking whole grains and beans is intimidating due to the time factor involved, consider two solutions at the opposite ends of the spectrum, pressure cooking and slow cooking. Pressure cooking comes with its own intimidating reputation, but modern pressure cookers are quite safe. Once you get past their "dangerous" reputation, you'll discover that they cook grains and beans in a fraction of the time of regular cooking; black beans normally take around 2 hours to cook whereas in a pressure cooker they are done in about 20 minutes. And if you forget to presoak your beans, you can still pressure cook them faster than regular cooking with a presoak. The time advantage is similar with grains; for example, you can pressure cook brown rice faster than cooking white rice in a regular pot. Pressure cooking also retains more nutrients in the finished food than does regular cooking.

With slow cooking, alternatively, you put your food into the crock in the morning and walk away. The food cooks gently under low heat through the day, and is ready for dinner. The cooking takes more time on the clock, but in terms of the time you have to put in preparing the meal, this can be a real convenience. Both pressure cooking and slow cooking have another advantage: they use less energy in cooking the food than normal stovetop methods.

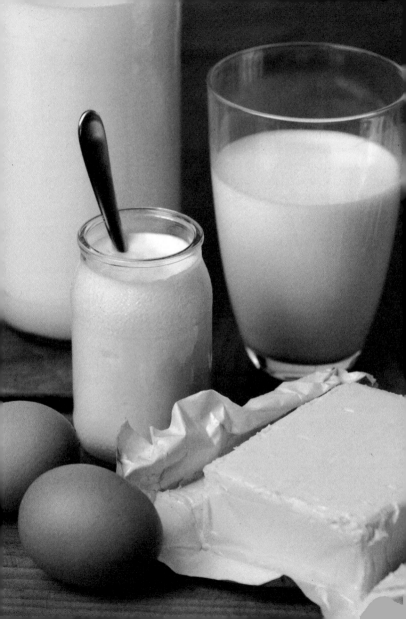

Chapter 4

MILK, CHEESE, AND YOGURT

It's not necessary to consume any dairy products to be healthy, but the National Dairy Council works hard to convince Americans otherwise. The trade organization behind the ubiquitous "Got Milk?" advertising campaign, the NDC is well funded and politically powerful. In 2004, the NDC used its influence to push the USDA into increasing their recommended servings of dairy from two to three per day for adults—a decision that had exactly nothing to do with health concerns. Rather, it was a calculated move to increase profits.

For many people, dairy products like ice cream, cheese, full-fat yogurt, and whole milk are comfort foods, but the levels of saturated fat and calories found within them mean they should be consumed in moderation. Also, never forget that the higher cost of organic dairy represents the true price of creating these products in a humane, healthy, and sustainable manner, while the reasons conventional dairy remains cheap are precisely the same reasons that it's bad for the environment, as well as human and animal health.

By savoring organic dairy products, and using them sparingly, you can stretch their value, enjoy them more, and feel better while you do.

Homogenization and Pasteurization

Almost all the milk available in grocery stores has been homogenized and pasteurized. Certain brands of organic milk are not homogenized, so the cream rises to the top and the container has to be shaken before drinking. To prevent this separation, the homogenization process essentially mixes the milk so strongly that the fatty cream particles stay suspended in the whey.

The pasteurization process was invented in order to prevent bacterial disease in dairy products—a considerable danger in the days before refrigeration—and involves heating milk to a temperature sufficient to destroy bacteria without being so hot that it ruins the flavor. The label "ultrapasteurized" means the milk was heated to an extremely high temperature, but only for one or two seconds. Unfortunately, no matter how it's accomplished, pasteurization destroys lactase, the enzyme that digests lactose, the sugary protein in milk. Many lactose-intolerant people suffer from the ailment precisely because of this missing lactase enzyme.

Health Concerns: Antibiotics and Growth Hormones

Cows given genetically modified recombinant bovine growth hormone (rBGH) produce a lot more milk, which in turn makes their milk artificially cheap. But this increased production also dilutes vitamin content, since each cow only has a finite amount of vitamins to contribute to her milk.

By treating dairy cows as machines and using rBGH to push output, conventional producers also expose their herds to udder infections, which are treated using antibiotics. These antibiotics enter the food supply and can lead to antibiotic resistance in humans. Constantly drinking low doses of antibiotics also destroys the beneficial "probiotic" bacteria in your digestive tract.

In contrast, the organic-foods movement addresses many of the problems that arise from applying industrial agribusiness methods to the dairy farm. For instance, all certified organic dairy products must meet the following standards: animals must be given organic feed, access to pasture, outdoor air, and sunlight, shade, and shelter; plus animals cannot be given hormones or antibiotics (except to treat disease, in which case their milk is removed from the food supply).

So why are all these precautions necessary? Critics allege that genetically modified recombinant bovine growth hormone causes human adolescents to experience puberty earlier, and leads to increased risks of certain cancers. But there are no conclusive scientific studies that prove or disprove these claims, which is why you'll see an asterisk on food labels that say "Produced without rBGH*" or "Milk from cows not given rBGH*," with the asterisk leading to a qualifying statement from the FDA that reads, "Milk produced without rBGH is not demonstrably different from milk produced with rBGH."

With or without an asterisk, organic dairies certainly represent a strong step in the right direction, but even "organic" cows often remain confined and are usually fed organic grain instead of grazing on their natural diet of grass. Whether raised for beef or dairy, grass-fed bovines are much healthier and better for the environment. Milk from cows raised on pasture is also higher in cancer-fighting conjugated linoleic acid (CLA), and the balance of essential fatty acids in the milk is in correct proportion for optimal health. Pastured milk also provides higher levels of calcium and vitamins A and E, since the lack of growth hormones leaves its vitamin content undiluted.

Goat's Milk

Goat's milk offers an attractive alternative to cow's milk, and is actually consumed by the majority of dairy users worldwide. Goats produce much less methane and other greenhouse gases when compared to cows, so choosing goat's milk is an effective way to reduce your carbon "foodprint." Homogenization isn't necessary for goat's milk, because the fat globules are smaller and remain suspended on their own. These smaller fat particles also allow for easier digestion, passing through the human digestive system in as little as half an hour—as opposed to cow's milk, which can require a full day.

Quicker, easier digestion lessens the feelings of indigestion and bloat that some people experience after consuming too much dairy food. Goat's milk also contains less lactose, making it tolerable for some people who are allergic to cow's milk, plus it has more vitamin A, B1, calcium, iron, and phosphorus.

The pH balance of goat's milk is alkaline, like mother's milk, while cow's milk is acidic. Dietary pH has effects on health, and most people's diets are too acidic. Eating more alkaline foods helps to balance your "inner ecology," a concept central to Chinese and holistic medicine.

Yogurt

Yogurt is milk that has been eaten and digested by colony-forming bacteria cultures. It has a much longer shelf life than milk, which makes going organic a more budget-friendly option. You can further budget on yogurt by purchasing the plain flavor and adding your own maple syrup, honey, or other sweetener, which will also cut down on the excess added sugars most flavored yogurt products contain. Adding your own fruit and granola instantly creates a pleasant, and healthy, breakfast or snack. Look for the "Live and Active Cultures" seal from the National Yogurt Association, or, better yet, use last week's leftover organic milk to create your own yogurt—a simple, fun, and rewarding project.

Cheese

Since cheese is basically solid fat, it's best enjoyed in moderation, or perhaps as a substitute for even more fattening desserts. As a reward for eating less cheese (and eliminating cheap imitation "cheese food" entirely), treat yourself to the best you can afford, and don't be afraid to try new varieties. Fine cheese is a great joy, and connoisseurs treasure the distinct flavors of sharp Cheddar, Brie, Gruyère, and Roquefort no less than lovers of fine wine value a good vintage.

Remember to always let cheese warm to room temperature before eating it. Avoid touching cheese with your fingers if you are going to wrap that section again and return it to the fridge, because your

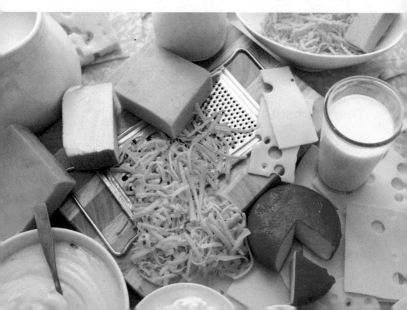

PSSSST—GOT ANY RAW DAIRY?

Raw milk is unpasteurized, unhomogenized whole milk straight from the cow's teat. Sounds delicious, but if you'd like to experience the nuances in taste present in all-natural milk, as well as its health benefits, you might have to break the law.

In many states it's illegal to even give away raw milk, so if you lack a backyard dairy cow, you'll have to seek out the raw milk underground. Sandor Ellix Katz covers the raw milk movement in his book, The Revolution Will Not Be Microwaved: America's Underground Food Movements (see the "Resources" section). He describes a dedicated community of milk connoisseurs who find loopholes in the regulations that prohibit raw milk distribution, arranging for members of private clubs to purchase a share of a cow or goat and share the output.

For more information about the health benefits of raw milk, visit the Weston A. Price Foundation at westonaprice.org.

hands can introduce bacteria that cause mold—though small patches of mold are harmless and can be cut off in any case.

Dairy Substitutes

Reducing dairy consumption is a good idea for any heavy user. Imitation products meant to mimic dairy can also provide much-needed substitutions for vegans or those with specific health concerns like lactose intolerance or milk allergies.

Nut milks and "not milks"

If you normally eat cereal for breakfast, all-natural nut milks make an excellent and nutritious substitute for cow's milk. Almond milk is commonly available, and it's easy to make your own too. Simply soak raw almonds overnight (or use a generous scoop of nut butter), then puree in a blender with plenty of water, and add a few drops of almond extract or honey. If you prefer smoother milk, strain it through cheesecloth.

Hemp milk offers an excellent compromise between grain- and nut-based "milks," since hemp milk tastes great and is also rich in omega-3s and other nutrients. The drawback is that it's not widely available and can be expensive. Minimally processed, organic rice and soy milks also make acceptable substitutes, but check the label to make sure they're not packed with added sweeteners.

For coffee, try a tiny bit of coconut milk, which you may find tastes even better than the cow's milk you're replacing. On the other hand, nondairy creamers are essentially—in the words of nutritionist Marion Nestle—"white, sweet, liquid margarines," i.e., "fake foods" that should be avoided.

Margarine

In its true form, margarine is an unattractive grayish white. Because of dairy-industry opposition, artificial yellow coloring wasn't allowed until the 1950s, when lawmakers—influenced by "Big Margarine" lobbyists—finally gave in and repealed the law that prevented fake "butter" from being artificially colored.

Margarine is whipped together mainly from soy oil, preservatives, and artificial flavorings, and costs much less than butter owing to the "miracle" of food technology. Currently, margarine is marketed as a health food, but there's no real evidence that it's any healthier than butter, especially considering recent revelations about the increased risks of disease caused by trans fats from partially hydrogenated oils. For those seeking to avoid butter based on allergies, or for vegans who avoid all dairy, Dr. Andrew Weil recommends Spectrum Spread in his book, *The Healthy Kitchen*.

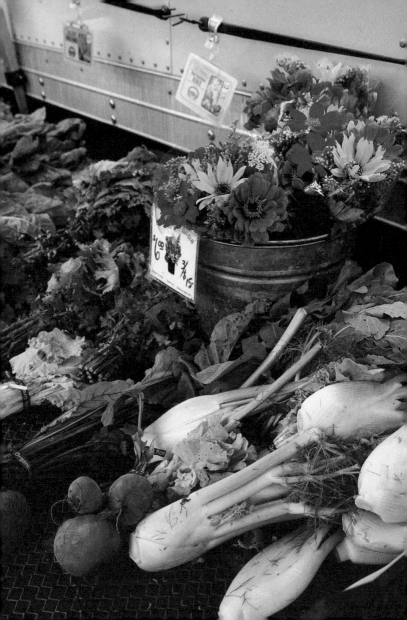

Chapter 5

VEGETABLES AND FRUITS

Adding seasonal, organic, local fruits and vegetables to your diet provides a sensory treat, while at the same time supporting the most environmentally friendly agriculture possible. Raw, pickled, sautéed, steamed, or roasted, vegetables bring a variety of flavors to a meal, while fruits offer up an irresistibly sweet treat that's perfect for breakfast, dessert, and snacks throughout a busy day. Best of all, studies show that people who eat five or more servings of fruits and vegetables daily may have half the cancer risk of people who eat only two servings, which makes this one food group where it's impossible to overdo it.

Ready to Eat

Watch the television commercials pushing fake foods like Toaster Strudels, Go-Gurt, and frozen dinner entrées, and the main selling point usually boils down to convenience. But what could be more convenient than biting into an apple, steaming some spinach, peeling a carrot, or munching on a carton of berries? Salads toss together in a minute, and most fruits and vegetables taste best, and provide their best nourishment, when enjoyed either raw or minimally cooked.

Prepared more elaborately, fruits and vegetables can also rival any dish as the height of fine dining, and make a satisfying stand-in for those seeking to either go vegetarian or simply eat less meat. For instance,

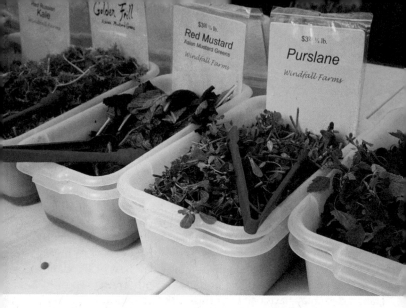

try replacing the chicken in your next batch of chicken Parmesan with thinly sliced and lightly fried eggplant instead, and see if anyone from your family complains. Odds are they'll ask for seconds instead!

Selecting Produce

Look for freshness, and remember that your best ally is your sense of smell. Fruit should smell ripe, lettuce should be crisp. Always look for intact leaves and stems; avoid wilted, dried out, or limp specimens. However, be aware that imperfections are natural, and slightly odd shapes or an occasional blemish shouldn't dissuade you from choosing a ripe fruit or veggie. Only chemicals, plastic wrapping, and protective fungicidal waxes make uniform, perfect, shiny produce possible.

Beware of pre-bagged salad mixes, "baby" carrots, or precut veggies or fruit salad. This minimal processing adds greatly to the cost of produce, increases chances for contamination, and requires plastic packaging. Bags of salad mix are injected with gases to keep leaves looking their best, and many of these prepared salads have traveled for weeks before they reach your cart.

Health Risks and Environmental Issues

Fruits and vegetables provide the base of an environmentally friendly diet. Choosing organic, local, seasonal varieties helps foster good health and sustainable agriculture.

Pesticides

While the federal government regulates which pesticides farmers can use and in what amounts, America's conventional agricultural system nonetheless requires the application of more than 1.2 billion pounds of chemical pesticides each year, according to the Pesticide Action Network (www.pesticideinfo.org), with their toxic residue ending up in our groundwater, on our food and, ultimately, under our skin. Excessive exposure to pesticides may increase your risk of cancer and hormone disruption. Collateral damage to the environment from pesticides includes runoff into waterways, which leads to destruction of aquatic life, birds, and other wild creatures.

Studies show that people who consistently eat organic fruits and vegetables have lower levels of pesticides in their bodies, which makes it important to buy organic as much as possible. Also, thoroughly wash fruits and vegetables before consuming them, particularly if you plan to eat the skin or other outer covering. Avoid buying conventional versions of fruits and vegetables that have thin or no skins, since these varieties absorb the most pesticides, like peaches, apples, sweet bell peppers, celery, nectarines, strawberries, cherries, lettuce, grapes (imported), pears, spinach, and potatoes. Conventional strawberries are especially worrisome because of the presence of methyl bromide, a known carcinogen and ozone-eroding chemical that is absorbed into the flesh of the berry so that it cannot be washed off.

Fruits and veggies carrying the least measurable contaminants include onions, avocadoes, sweet corn (frozen), pineapples, mango, sweet peas (frozen), asparagus, kiwi, bananas, cabbage, broccoli, and eggplant. You can save money by buying conventional versions of these fruits and vegetables.

Check foodnews.org, a project of the Environmental Working Group, for updated pesticide advisories.

Fertilizer

Over time, cultivating conventional of just one type of fruit or vegetable ("monocropping") degrades farmland fertility, leading to increasingly intense applications of chemical fertilizers. Derived from petroleum, these synthetic fertilizers contribute to climate change. Excess nitrogen from synthetic fertilizers used to boost yields of conventional fruits and vegetables contaminates our surface and ground waters and has even created a massive "dead zone" in the Gulf of Mexico, where nitrogen-fed algal blooms choke out all other aquatic life. Unless individuals, governments, and, most importantly, industrial farmers begin to make necessary changes, this situation will continue to worsen.

Buying organic fruits and vegetables helps preserve your health, the soil, and the environment, particularly if these products are grown on farms that incorporate sustainable farming processes like crop rotation, cover crops, natural pest controls, and no-till farming.

Heirloom Produce

Today, many species of food plants have been hybridized for various reasons, usually to improve disease resistance, taste, or yield. Using the traditional techniques of cross-pollination and selection, farmer-breeders have always manipulated plant genetics to improve plant varieties in ways that suit their own purposes. Specific fruits or veggies described as "heirloom" are open-pollinated varieties (i.e., can reproduce themselves from seed) that have been passed down for many generations, often within an ethnic population, tribe, or family. Heirloom tomatoes have once again become very popular among home gardeners and in farmers markets, along with traditional Southwestern blue corn and purple potatoes. Different shapes, colors, and tastes distinguish heirlooms, and along with this diversity of form come unique traits that are worth saving for future eaters, like resistance to diseases or pests or adaptability to a specific growing region (or to uncertain climatic conditions).

Whereas heirloom varieties are often more local and specialized, and take a while to adapt to a new home, commercial hybrids are designed to grow and yield relatively well in a wide range of conditions. And while heirlooms also offer gardeners and small farmers other

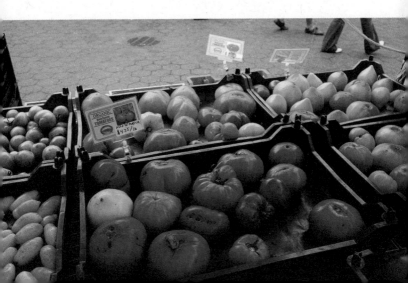

benefits, such as a long harvest season, hybrids are usually bred for large commercial growers who want to harvest a crop all at one time, often with the use of machinery. Hybrids have also been developed with other needs of industrial agriculture in mind: tough skins for shipability; extended shelf life; multiple insect and disease resistance (which is required for large monocrop plantings); and uniformity of size. Rarely, if ever, are taste and nutrition the aims of the modern agribusiness plant breeder.

Choosing Organic

Organic produce isn't always more expensive. When in season, the price of organic fruits and vegetables can be equal to or less than the "conventional" choices. Consider reducing your budget for meat and dairy—with their high costs and large carbon footprints—and putting the money you save toward healthier organic fruits and veggies. You'll be sending a powerful message to America's agribusinesses about the kind of food you want to eat, and the kind of world you want to live in.

Choosing Local

When fruits and vegetables grown all over the country get processed at a centralized location, the dangers of tampering, accidental contamination, and supply-chain disruption become magnified, especially once this produce has been redistributed across the country, as we have seen with recent scares over bacterial contamination of spinach, jalapenos, and peanuts. Local distribution, on the other hand, ensures less of a widespread health hazard should contamination occur, as well as relative ease in tracing any problem to its source.

Beyond health security, buying local fruits and veggies means fewer "food miles" are traveled between the field and your plate, thus ensuring reduced greenhouse gas emissions. Most importantly, seasonal, local fruits and vegetables will be fresher and tastier, hence more nutritious and satisfying than food transported a thousand miles in a cold-chain refrigerated system that includes intermediate truck stops at the warehouse, distributor, and grocery store.

Choosing Seasonal

Buying fresh fruits and vegetables when they are in season costs less, since large quantities of these highly perishable foods hit the market all at once, lowering prices. Preserve this bounty by pickling cucumbers, canning tomatoes, jarring your own applesauce, and drying almost any variety of fruit. Also, consider purchasing pounds of nectarines and extra baskets of berries during the summer, at the height of their seasonal flavor, and freezing them to enjoy in smoothies throughout the year.

Assuming that you have a freezer in your home, keep in mind that it will work most efficiently when at or near capacity. Choose the size of freezer that best matches your individual needs (or no freezer at all), and then plan carefully to keep it full with the fewest trips to the store.

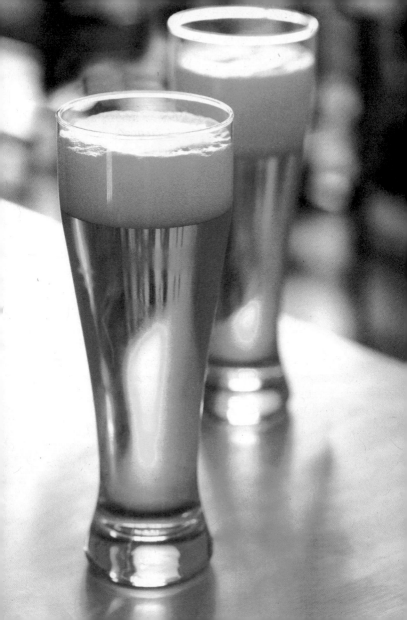

Chapter 6

BEER, WINE, AND SPIRITS

Beer, wine, and spirits enjoy a history with humankind that's as long as agriculture itself. Valued as a way to preserve and store harvests (not to mention cop a buzz), every culture in the world has its own traditional fermented brews, from sake (rice wine) in Japan to *chicha* (corn beer) in South America. Even during our hunting-and-gathering days, humans enjoyed the miracle of fermented honey, known as mead—the world's oldest alcoholic beverage.

Next time you sit down to enjoy a healthy meal featuring whole grains, organic beans, and local veggies, reward yourself by washing it all down with a glass of organic or local beer or wine. Red wine has a remarkable amount of antioxidants, and drinking alcohol in moderation (no more than two drinks per day!) contributes to better heart health. The main environmental issues to consider with beer, wine, and spirits are the same as with other foods: how and where were they produced? Strict vegetarians and vegans should also know that certain beers and wines use animal products as clarifying agents in the fermentation process.

Beer

After more than a thousand years of traditional brewing, the ingredients used to create high-quality beer remain relatively simple: water, hops, malted barley, and yeast. Replace barley with wheat and you get Hefeweizen, or "white" (wit) beers. Also, keep in mind that national, corporate brands like Budweiser, Coors, and Miller use adjuncts like corn and rice, resulting in light-colored, watery beers with a lower alcohol content and little taste.

Fortunately, America's once proud tradition of regional and local breweries has been experiencing a major renaissance, which means you can easily find a favorite beer that's brewed close to home, including often an organic brand. Organic beers fall under the same rules that govern organic food production, so any six-pack bearing the familiar USDA seal signifies that the brew is made of organic hops and grain. However, owing to smaller consumer demand for organic beers, the hops and barley used may have been imported from New Zealand, Germany, or elsewhere overseas, resulting in a somewhat less "local" libation.

Conventional cultivation of hops often includes a heavy reliance on synthetic fertilizers and high levels of fungicides because of the plant's susceptibility to downy mildew. More than 70 percent of U.S. hops are grown in Washington's Yakima Valley, an important watershed for endangered wild salmon, so reducing harmful chemical run-off is a worthwhile goal supported by your organic beer purchases.

Whether you imbibe locally, organically, or both, give thanks that conscientious consumers now have a choice that reflects their values. The microbrewery revolution that began in the 1980s, along with the success of organic foods, proves that when given an option, people will choose a unique, high-quality experience of food and drink that reflects the culture of where they live. Local beers also help improve your "food mileage," since quaffing the output of your neighborhood microbrewery reduces the need for trucking heavy beer bottles and kegs. Many small breweries also make use of "growlers," reusable glass jugs that can be filled up by loyal customers again and again, often at a more affordable price than six-packs.

If you consistently drink beer at home, especially in a shared house with several roommates, consider buying or building your own "kegerator," a customized fridge that keeps a barrel cold, with taps built in to dispense perfect pints. Using kegs saves money, and it also eliminates the need to manufacture and recycle a new glass bottle for every twelve ounces of beer.

Creative, economical people should also try brewing their own beer or making their own wine or hard cider. It's not as hard as you think, and there's nothing more local!

Wine

Conventional vineyards use lots of pesticides, herbicides, fumigants, and synthetic fertilizers. Thirsty grapes can also require a lot of water, creating a serious issue in arid climates. Happily, the movement toward sustainable viticulture gains strength each year, particularly in California, which supplies the United States with 90 percent of its wine.

According to the *Sonoma Index-Tribune*, the wine industry's cumulative use-intensity for pesticides declined by 84 percent in Napa County and 46 percent in Sonoma County in the years between 1993 and 2000, a welcome trend that reflects the growing sustainability movement on the West Coast. Many wineries have also begun increasing the health of their soil and preventing soil erosion by planting cover crops, adding companion plants to encourage beneficial insects, and aggressively conserving water.

Wines labeled "100% Organic" must be made from organically grown grapes, cannot have any added sulfites, and must list the certifying agency. If the label says, "Made with Organic Grapes," (or "Organically Grown Grapes") the wine may have had some sulfites added. Biodynamic vineyards go well beyond organic, making wines in tune with natural rhythms and larger cosmic forces, while nurturing vines on vital, living soil. Wineries focused on sustainability include Frey, Bonterra, Coturri, and Benziger.

Sulfites in Wine

Sulfites occur naturally in wine, but in trace amounts. Most winemakers add extra sulfur dioxide to preserve wine from oxidation, thus maintaining its flavor, aroma, and clarity for years. Sulfites also are used in dried fruit, fruit concentrates, jellies, jams, syrups, pizza dough, frozen potatoes, and many other products.

Sulfite content became a labeling issue for wines because sulfites are a known allergen. Otherwise, sulfites have no known negative effects on the environment or health. Very few people are allergic to sulfites, but quite a few folks are sensitive to them—especially asthmatics—which means consuming sulfites can lead to heartburn, hives, and other adverse but nonthreatening reactions.

For a wine to be considered 100 percent organic, there must be no added sulfites, and the total sulfite content must be less than 20 parts per million (ppm). If you see "Sulfite-Free" on a bottle, the levels are so low as to be undetectable. Bottles labeled "Made from Organic Grapes" contain added sulfites, but typically at levels lower than conventional wine.

Vegan Beers and Wines

For vegans, minute quantities of animal-derived ingredients in beer and wine like albumin, casein, charcoal, glyceryl monostearate, isinglass, gelatin, and pepsin create major concerns. Used to protect taste and color or to reduce the foam in beer, these agents work as electrostatic magnets that attract unwanted matter from the bottom of the tanks. It's impossible to know where these ingredients might show up since beer and wine have no labeling requirements, but a little Internet research reveals which brands are truly vegan.

Animal-derived fining agents are more commonly used in beers produced in the UK and Ireland. (Guinness uses isinglass, which is derived from fish bladders, as a fining agent.) Samuel Smith's beers, also from the UK, are completely vegan, so enjoy an Oatmeal Stout instead of your Guinness if use of these fining agents disturbs you. These animal-derived fining agents are rarely used by brewers in the United States, Germany, or Belgium, where breweries and wineries typically use sterile filtration that removes all traces of these agents from the finished drink.

Many vegan wines are now made with clay, diatomaceous earth, or carbon as fining agents. Google "vegan wine and beer" for more information.

Spirits

After the repeal of Prohibition in 1933, most distilling and production of spirits was taken over by large companies. Lately, however, in the wake of successful organic wineries and microbreweries, artisanal spirits have started appearing in the United States. These smaller distilleries focus on high-quality ingredients and painstaking craftsmanship to create new, unique libations. Many of these businesses also commit to using recyclable, eco-friendly packaging.

Organic vodkas are the fastest growing and easiest to find, with a number of brands debuting recently, such as Square One Organic Vodka, Crop Vodka, Prairie Organic Vodka, TRU Organic Spirits, and Vodka 14. The Organic Spirits Company offers certified organic whiskey under the name "Highland Harvest," as well as gin and rum. The tequila brand 4 Copas is made from certified organic agave plants.

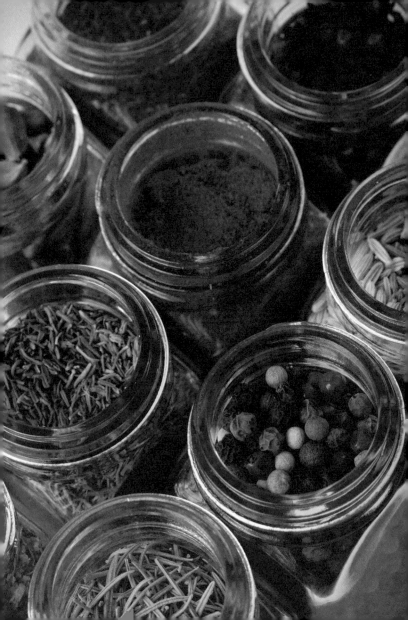

Chapter 7

COFFEE, TEA, SWEETS, AND SPICES

Many exotic goods that originate in distant lands were considered luxuries one hundred years ago, but today we take them thoroughly for granted. In our modern, global market for food, the way we buy and transport imported items like coffee, tea, chocolate, sugar, and spices deeply affects cultures and ecosystems all over the world, which means we must take responsibility for the consequences—pro and con—of our purchasing decisions. Exercising food mindfulness means being extra appreciative of imported luxuries: for example, the next time you drink a cup of Indian tea, imagine every person that had a hand in bringing the experience to your breakfast table.

Imported foods carrying the "Fair Trade" label have been certified for adherence to fair-labor standards and benign environmental effects. Approximately 80 percent of Fair Trade–certified farmers do not use synthetic fertilizers or chemical pest and weed controls on their fields, and the small, family farms and locally owned cooperatives that participate in these progressive programs are more likely to be effective caretakers of their land than multinational corporations. Fair trade also assures growers of a more sustainable floor price for their crop.

Direct trade takes this concept even further, with companies in consumer countries establishing direct relationships with grower cooperatives. These arrangements often ensure a better-than-fair-trade price, plus, in some cases, profit sharing and assistance for local farmers to improve conditions in what are often poor rural communities.

Coffee

Faraway countries that produce luxurious commodities are often extremely impoverished and do not regulate pesticide use as the United States does. Toxic chemicals (like DDT) banned in the United States are still in use elsewhere around the world. Conventional coffee is produced using tons of pesticides and herbicides, often on easily eroded land where fertility is lost after only a few growing seasons. New, high-yielding varieties of coffee plants have been bred to grow in full sun, meaning that large forests are chopped down to make way for monocropped fields.

Coffees labeled "Shade-Grown" or "Bird-Friendly" are cultivated under partial forest canopy, preserving habitat that supports some birds and wildlife. The Rainforest Alliance certifies both products that meet their goals of long-term sustainability of tropical rainforests and occupations that provide the human inhabitants of these ecologically precious places with a living wage.

Green, Black, and Herbal Teas

Drinking tea is preferable to coffee for a variety of health reasons: caffeine is damaging in a number of different ways, and many people are addicted to coffee, making it difficult to give up cold turkey. Coffee is hard on the kidneys and liver, and the stimulating effect of caffeine is caused by the body working to eliminate this "poison" as quickly as possible.

Green and black teas have protective antioxidants, and while tea leaves contain more caffeine than coffee beans, the steeped brew doesn't contain as much as a cup of joe. Green tea also contains amino acids that produce a less nerve-wracking wake-up, which is why many people who are sensitive to coffee prefer tea. Try a relaxing tea ceremony in the mornings, gearing yourself up for a calm, but lively and productive day. Herbal teas have a host of medicinal effects that are beyond the scope of this book, but check out the Internet for more information. Loose-leaf teas are often cheaper than packaged teas in baggies, and all you need is a reusable metal tea ball.

Sugar and Sweeteners

Massive oversweetening of the American diet through processed foods and soft drinks causes childhood diabetes and contributes to obesity. Excessive sugar in a child's diet has been linked to aggressive behavior, as well as difficulty holding concentration. Sugar is best used in very small amounts, not just because of its health effects, but also because of its disastrous legacy of labor abuse and environmental devastation. In Florida, sugarcane cultivation is linked to pollution and heavy water use that threatens the Everglades. As with any other foods, choose organic, fair-trade sugar, and use much less of it.

Avoid artificial sweeteners, those insidious "fake foods" that are sneaked into innumerable industrial food products. The best rule of thumb is to reject any product with unpronounceable ingredients or any "white powder" substance. Like hard drugs, sugar, Splenda, and saccharine are refined and adulterated, and items like sorbitol and maltitol cannot be digested. High-fructose corn syrup, created as a by-product of government-subsidized cheap corn, is included in a ridiculous amount of packaged foods.

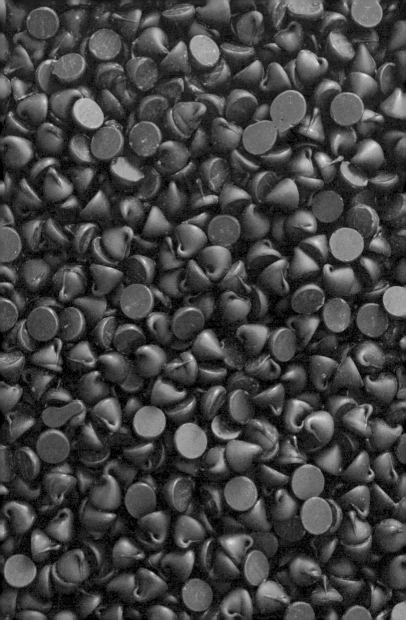

More sustainable, natural sweeteners include real maple syrup (not maple-flavored corn syrup), honey, agave, molasses, and brown rice syrup. You can use these sweets in recipes; and when craving a sugary snack, satisfy yourself with dried or fresh fruit, juice, or a smoothie instead.

Chocolate and Cocoa

Biochemically speaking, eating chocolate produces an effect similar to being in love, a mood enhancement that comes courtesy of the moderate amount of caffeine and theobromines that are present, especially in dark chocolate. Unfortunately, cocoa trees only produce for about twenty-five years; once the land is exhausted, growers move on to virgin land. And so, our love affair with cocoa—which, when combined with milk, sugar, and butter becomes silky chocolate—indirectly deforests vast areas of equatorial land. Also, commercial cocoa production in Africa commonly uses child labor, often in conditions that equate to modern-day slavery.

Sourcing organic, fair-trade chocolate and cocoa is the best way for consumers to send a signal to producers that these conditions are unacceptable. Cacao, like coffee, can be shade-grown in a mixed forest-garden planting that's actually environmentally beneficial; it doesn't need to be grown on large plantations. In fact, many high-end chocolates are now made with single-estate cacao beans, so it is easier to trace not just the origin, but also the environmental and social factors involved in its production.

While it's not always true that more expensive chocolate is better for the earth, you should do your homework and go for the good stuff—just eat a lot less of it. Like wine and beer, consuming small amounts of cocoa has health benefits, but there's still a lot of fat in chocolate. Treat it like cheese or alcohol—it's good in moderation.

Spices

Keep your eyes peeled for fresh herbs at farmers markets, and cultivate your own whenever possible. Potted basil, thyme, sage, and oregano are beautiful and easy to grow and use, and you can harvest bold flavors that will beat any dried-out version from the pantry.

Salt, the world's most commonly used condiment and food additive, makes food sparkle with flavor when the right amount is added. While all table salt is sodium chloride, not all salt is equal. Refined table salt loses all flavor except bitterness after being dried at extremely high temperatures and bleached. When iodine (an essential human nutrient) is added, all other minerals are lost completely. On the other hand, Celtic sea salt is skimmed off the top of tidal pools and dried in the sun, allowing it to retain more than eighty minerals and a pleasant taste. Many different kinds of salt are available, including kosher salt, Himalayan crystal salt, and salts from other exotic locales such as Hawaii or India. Experiment with different salts to find one (or more) that you like, and avoid overly salted junk foods.

Pepper, while just as common as salt, really shines when dried, whole peppercorns are ground before being added to foods. The difference in flavor between freshly ground pepper and pre-ground is astounding. Black, white, and green peppercorns come from the same plant, but are harvested at varying degrees of ripeness for variations in flavor.

When seeking out cumin, turmeric, ginger, caraway, nutmeg, cinnamon, or any other spice, look for a certified organic and/or fair-trade label. Conventional spice production uses either irradiation or carcinogenic chemicals like ethylene oxide or methyl bromide to sterilize spices and remove any biological contaminants.

Organic spice producers use none of these industrial, chemical methods, preferring instead to use steam or carbon dioxide to sterilize

spices. Companies like Frontier and ForesTrade have forged partnerships with spice farmers in foreign lands to improve their wages and
sponsor environmental stewardship.

Even though spices constitute a small part of a meal, it can be argued
that these miniscule amounts of spice can make or break a dish—just
a tad too much cayenne pepper can heatedly illustrate this point! For
the best flavor and value, chefs advise purchasing whole spices, and
grinding or toasting them as needed. Storing dried, pre-ground spices for more than a few months can leave them stale and flavorless.

Oils

High-quality, cold-pressed, pure oils build the foundation of good
cooking.

Avoid refined oils, which are chemically treated by using a solvent to
extract oil from seeds (or nuts), then bleached, steamed, and clarified,
removing any flavor or nutritional value, and resulting in an odorless,
tasteless product best used to lubricate rusty hinges.

Seek out fine, estate-bottled olive oils to drizzle over cooked veggies
or to make salad dressings, and use cheaper extra virgin or pure olive
oil for sautéing. Olive oil is monounsaturated, which makes it a "good
fat" when consumed in moderation, not to mention one of the pil-
lars of the famous Mediterranean diet touted by doctors and nutri-
tionists. Canola oil is also highly recommended, along with sesame,
safflower, and sunflower. As always, seek out organic oils whenever
possible.

Store oils in the fridge, especially if you won't be using them immediately. Oils may become "cloudy" when cooled, a normal chemical re-
action that's easily reversed by returning them to room temperature.

Cut Flowers

Mother's Day and Valentine's Day, along with many other celebrations, bring family, friends, and lovers bearing bright bouquets. These cut flowers hide a disturbing chemical legacy behind their blooms and fragrance, especially because regulations intended to limit applications of pesticides to edible items do not apply to inedible decorations. Flower plantations, many located in equatorial locations, expose workers, local communities, and florists to toxic pollution. Give a sustainable, sweet-smelling gift, and source your flowers from local farmers or from organicbouquet.com.

WHAT TO LOOK FOR ON IMPORTED GOODS

Fair Trade. Some produce cannot be grown locally, including tropical fruit and everyone's favorite drugs of choice, coffee and sugar. Cacao beans and many spices also originate in equatorial locales, and while some locavores eschew these items, others allow a limited quota for consumption of exotic luxuries. "Fair trade" labels indicate that the coffee, tea, herbs, chocolate, sugar, spices, honey, rice, flowers, and fresh or dried fruits in question were produced according to standards of just labor practices and sustainable environmental conditions.

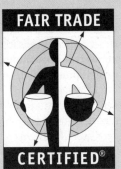

RESOURCES

Further Reading

Annemarie Colbin. *Food and Healing*. New York, NY.: Ballantine Books, 1986.

Sandor Ellix Katz. *The Revolution Will Not Be Microwaved: Inside America's Underground Food Movements*. White River Junction, VT: Chelsea Green, 2006.

Marion Nestle. *What to Eat: A Shopper's Guide down the Aisles*, New York, NY: North Point Press, 2007.

Michael Pollan. *Omnivore's Dilemna*. New York, NY: Penguin, 2006.

Elizabeth Rogers, and Thomas M. Kostigen. *The Green Book,* New York, NY: Three Rivers Press, 2007.

Alisa Smith and J. B. MacKinnon. *Plenty: One Man, One Woman and a Raucous Year of Eating Locally,* New York, NY: Harmony Books, 2007.

Ann Vilensis. *Kitchen Literacy*, Washington, DC: Island Press, 2007.

Vegetarian Cookbooks
Nava Atlas. *The Vegetarian 5-Ingredient Gourmet*. New York, NY: Broadway Books, 2001.

Peter Berley and Melissa Clark. *Fresh Food Fast*, New York, NY: Regan Books, 2004.

Matthew Kenney and Sarma Melngailis. *Raw Food/Real World*. New York, NY: Regan Books, 2006.

Flexitarian Cookbooks
Andrew Weil and Rosie Daley. *The Healthy Kitchen*. New York, NY: Alfred A. Knopf, 2003.

Jay Weinstein. *Ethical Gourmet*, New York, NY: Broadway Books, 2006.

On the Internet

Food and Environment
www.ethicurean.com. "Being an Ethicurean means simply trying to 'chew the right thing,'" and this blog updates conscious eaters about food policy, safety, and news, plus cooking, eating, and humor.

www.foodnews.org. Compiled by the Environmental Working Group, this site updates the "Dirty Dozen," that is, the foods most contaminated by pesticide residues. Also has information on their methodology for monitoring residues, plus tips to reduce your exposure.

Local Food
www.eatwellguide.org. "Eat Well Guide® is a free online directory of thousands of family farms, restaurants, and other outlets for fresh, locally grown food in the US and Canada."

www.localharvest.org. "LocalHarvest is America's #1 organic and local food Web site. We maintain a definitive and reliable "living" public nationwide directory of small farms, farmers markets, and other local food sources."

www.localfork.com. "Local Fork is an online community providing the tools to stimulate grassroots local food networks. Local Fork is the first Web site where local food consumers, buyers, and producers can fully collaborate, network, buy, sell, advertise, and find needed services."

www.foodroutes.org. "We are a national non-profit dedicated to reintroducing Americans to their food, the seeds it grows from, the farmers who produce it, and the routes that carry it from the fields to our tables."

Organic Food

www.organicconsumers.org "The OCA represents over 850,000 members, subscribers and volunteers, including several thousand businesses in the natural foods and organic marketplace. Our US and international policy board is broadly representative of the organic, family farm, environmental, and public interest community."

www.ams.usda.gov/nop. This is the government Web site for the National Organic Program.

Meat and Animal Issues

www.animalwelfareapproved.org. Animal Welfare Approved label program intended to inform consumers that their livestock was handled according to a set of standards that embodies "a philosophy of respect that provides animals on the farm with the environment, housing and diet they need to engage in essential instinctive behaviors, thereby promoting physiological and psychological health and well-being."

www.certifiedhumane.com. "The Certified Humane Raised and Handled® program is a certification and labeling program that is the only animal welfare label requiring the humane treatment of farm animals from birth through slaughter. The goal of the program is to improve the lives of farm animals by driving consumer demand for kinder and more responsible farm animal practices."

www.eatwild.com. "Your source for safe, healthy, natural and nutritious grass-fed beef, lamb, goats, bison, poultry, pork, dairy and other wild edibles."

Fish and Seafood

www.vitalchoice.com. "We seek to support our customers' well being, so Vital Choice will offer only the purest wild seafood possible: fish and shellfish that grow in the wild environment to which they are so superbly adapted, free of the antibiotics, pesticides, synthetic coloring agents, and genetically modified organisms (GMOs) used commonly in fish farms."

www.msc.org. "With experts we developed standards for sustainable fishing and seafood traceability. They ensure that MSC-labelled seafood comes from, and can be traced back to, a sustainable fishery."

www.mbayaq.org. Monterey Bay Aquarium site, the source for seafood wallet cards.

Wine and Beer

www.theorganicwinecompany.com. Source for earth-friendly wines along with resources about sustainable viticulture.

www.ottercreekbrewing.com. "One of the nation's original certified organic breweries, Wolaver's is committed to producing the best beer in the most ecologically sound way. Our craft ales are brewed using the finest organic malts, hops, our special house yeast, and pure Vermont water."

Coffee, Tea, Sweets, and Spices

www.transfairusa.org. "TransFair USA enables sustainable development and community empowerment by cultivating a more equitable global trade model that benefits farmers, workers, consumers, industry and the earth. We achieve our mission by certifying and promoting Fair Trade products."

www.greenpeople.org. "World's largest directory of eco-friendly and holistic health products."

Cooking

www.epicurious.com. Recipe search engine—just type in your ingredients, and a new dish pops up!

www.fastcooking.ca/pressurecookers/cookingtimes_pressure_cooker.php. For an extensive list of pressure cooking times.

www.vegetariantimes.com. Online magazine and resource for vegetarians, including recipe database.

Gardening

www.communitygardening.org. "The Mission of the American Community Gardening Association is to build community by increasing and enhancing community gardening and greening across the United States and Canada." Search for community gardens near you.

www.yougrowgirl.com. "You Grow Girl was launched by Gayla Trail in February 2000 and has grown into a thriving online community that speaks to a new kind of gardener, seeking to redefine the modern world relationship to plants. This contemporary, laid-back approach to gardening places equal importance on environmentalism, style, affordability, art, and humour."

THE CHELSEA GREEN GUIDES

Chelsea Green's new *Green Guides* are perfect tutors for individuals or businesses looking to green-up their knowledge. Each compact, value-priced guide is packed with tips that will improve the environment and your finances.

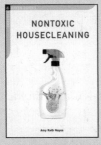

NONTOXIC HOUSECLEANING
AMY KOLB NOYES
9781603582032
$7.95

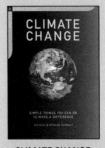

CLIMATE CHANGE:
*Simple Things You Can Do
to Make a Difference*
JON CLIFT and AMANDA CUTHBERT
9781603581066
$7.95

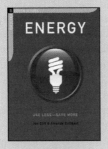

ENERGY:
Use Less—Save More
JON CLIFT and AMANDA CUTHBERT
9781933392721
$7.95

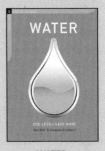

WATER:
Use Less—Save More
JON CLIFT and AMANDA CUTHBERT
9781933392738
$7.95

Slim enough to fit in a kitchen or desk drawer, you'll return to
the *Green Guides* frequently for concise, sage advice.

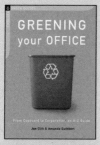

GREENING YOUR OFFICE
JON CLIFT and AMANDA CUTHBERT
9781933392998
$7.95

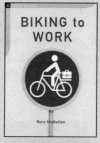

BIKING TO WORK
RORY MCMULLAN
9781933392981
$7.95

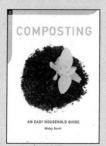

COMPOSTING:
An Easy Household Guide
NICKY SCOTT
9781933392745
$7.95

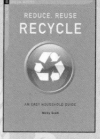

REDUCE, REUSE, RECYCLE:
An Easy Household Guide
NICKY SCOTT
9781933392752
$7.95

For more information or to request a catalog,
visit **www.chelseagreen.com** or call toll-free **(800) 639-4099**.

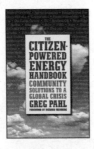
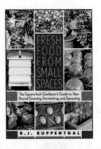
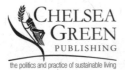